SECOND EDITION

Manual for IV Therapy Procedures

Shila R. Channell, RN, MSN, PhD

Medical Economics Books
Oradell, NJ 07649

Library of Congress Cataloging in Publication Data

Channell, Shila R.
   Manual for IV therapy procedures.

   Spine title: IV therapy procedures.
   Bibliography: p.
   Includes index.
   1. Intravenous therapy—Outlines, syllabi, etc.
I. Title.   II. Title: IV therapy procedures.   III. Title:
Manual for I.V. therapy procedures.   IV. Title: I.V.
therapy procedures.   [DNLM: 1. Infusions,
Parenteral—handbooks.   WB   39   C458m]
RM170.C46   1984   615.8'55   84-9367
ISBN 0-87489-370-4

Design by Penny Seldin
Cover photograph by Stephen Munz

ISBN 0-87489-370-4

Medical Economics Company Inc.
Oradell, New Jersey 07649

Printed in the United States of America

Table of contents

Preface

Intravenous therapy is playing an ever-larger role in health care. But when I looked for a text to adopt in my own classes, I found an incredible shortage of useful training materials. In response to that shortage, I compiled this manual for my students. Because I was instructing emergency medical technicians as well as students and nurses, I wanted the manual to be flexible enough to apply to emergencies in the field as well as the hospital setting. And, because I have taught IV therapy in different locales, I wanted to make the basic principles and practice understandable and assimilable into IV training programs everywhere. Finally, because I wanted it to be easy to use both as a text and as a refresher, I cast it in outline format.

Any invasive procedure breaks down the body's natural defense mechanisms and is a potential cause of infection. It is the responsibility of everyone involved in IV therapy to understand the care of the infusion site and equipment. It is equally important to recognize danger signals and take measures to prevent problems that can arise with patients and their infusion systems. Therefore, this manual presents guidelines to the principles as well as the practice of IV therapy and infection control.

Publisher's notes

Shila R. Channell, RN, MSN, PhD, brings to this outline guide a wealth of education and experience in intravenous therapy and infection control. She is presently director of nursing for Home Care America, Washington, D.C., and was formerly director of Infusion Services at the University of California, Davis Medical Center in Sacramento, California, and supervisor of the IV Therapy Department at Sinai Hospital, Baltimore, Maryland.

Prior to her position at Sinai, she was nurse epidemiologist at Harford Memorial Hospital, Havre de Grace, Maryland. She was also a member of the faculties of Harford Community College and Cecil Community College in Maryland, and was on staff at the American River College in California and the University of Central California. She has served as instructor in IV Therapy for the Harford County and Cecil County (Maryland) volunteer ambulance corps and the Emergency Medical Technicians program in California, and has taught the principles and practice of IV therapy to numerous RNs, LVNs, nursing students, paramedics, and technicians.

In addition to her other responsibilities, Dr. Channell has served as chairman of the Standards

Committee of the National Intravenous Therapy Association (1977-1978), president of the association's Chesapeake chapter (1978-1979), vice president of the Northern Maryland Association of Practitioners in Infection Control (1978-1979), and president of the Sacramento Valley Chapter of NITA (1983).

Dr. Channell was admitted to Sigma Theta Tau (national honor society for nurses) in 1983, and that same year was honored and presented with an award by the University of Central California for her contribution to excellence in medical education for the state of California.

Acknowledgments

My deepest love and appreciation go to my loving and patient husband, Stephen, for his support, encouragement, illustrations, and unwavering assistance in making this second edition a reality.

Gratitude also goes to those listed below for their contributions and assistance in making this second edition a better, more inclusive and effective manual:

Nabil Musallam, MS, RPh, Director, Pharmacy Department, University of California, Davis Medical Center, Sacramento, for critiquing of and additions to Chapters 11, 12, and 13.

Ray Howard, New Castle, California, and the University of California, Davis Medical Center, Sacramento, for the photography.

Margaret Sellers, RN, Sacramento, for critiquing of Chapter 20.

CHAPTER **1**

Introduction

A. PURPOSES OF IV INFUSION

- ▶ Administer medications, especially those needed to take effect quickly
- ▶ Supply nourishment, fluids, and electrolytes to body tissues
- ▶ Restore blood volume and correct deficiencies in blood components
- ▶ Stimulate the circulation in cases of shock and vascular collapse
- ▶ Maintain a line to the venous circulation of the patient
- ▶ Measure central venous pressure and blood gases if arterial blood isn't available
- ▶ Provide a pathway for anesthetics
- ▶ Obtain blood specimens (phlebotomy)
- ▶ Provide venous access for diagnostic exams (IVP, scans, etc.).

B. CHOICE OF METHOD

There are three basic ways to enter a vein. Choice depends on IV devices available, specific indications for use of IV route, and expertise.

1. Cutdown

Cutdown is surgical exposure of a vein. It's done when no surface veins are available for entry with a needle. The catheter is threaded directly into the exposed vein.

2. Catheter-through-needle

This device, or CTN, is used to enter large, deep veins such as the subclavian, jugular, or femoral (see Figure 1-1).

3. Catheter-over-needle and winged needle

The catheter-over-needle (CON) and winged needle (Figures 1-2 and 1-3) are used to enter peripheral veins. Peripheral venipuncture is by far the most common technique. It involves less trauma to patients, is less likely to create problems, is more convenient, and takes less time than a CTN or a surgical cutdown.

> ***a. Special advantages of the CON.*** With this device, the needle is entirely removed and disposed of after venipuncture. Because a catheter is flexible, not rigid like a needle, and no sharp needle is left in the vein, the risk of complications is greatly reduced, especially if the patient is active. Another advantage: The puncture in the vein is exactly the same size as the catheter, since the catheter enters the vein over the needle. This reduces the possibility of blood or fluid leakage around the venipuncture site. A CON is generally preferable to a needle.

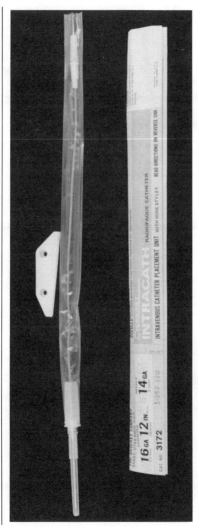

Figure 1-1 Catheter-through-needle (CTN) device

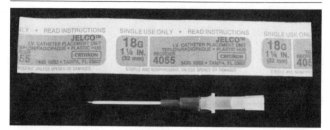

Figure 1-2 Catheter-over-needle (CON) device

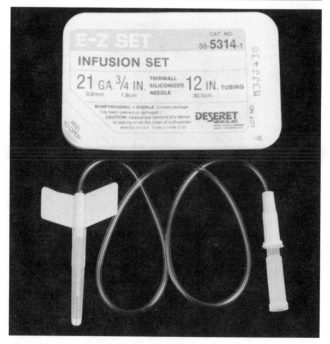

Figure 1-3 Winged infusion set

b. Special advantage of the winged needle.
With improvements in materials and
manufacturing methods, this device is being
increasingly supplanted by the CON.
However, a winged needle is still preferred
when it's necessary to use a very short or
small vein.

C. ASEPTIC TECHNIQUE

Whether a vein is entered by cutdown, by CTN, or
peripherally, except in critical emergencies, aseptic
technique must be used in preparing and
maintaining the injection site, and inserting the
intravenous device.

CHAPTER 2

The circulation

Veins present the most accessible route for parenteral therapy and nutrition, because they're abundant and easy to locate. Knowledge of the anatomy and physiology of veins and arteries will give you a sense of discrimination in choosing veins and help decrease trauma to patients.

A. THE CIRCULATORY SYSTEM

The body's circulatory system has two main subdivisions: cardiopulmonary and systemic.

1. The cardiopulmonary system

This system is not used for intravenous therapy, but it's helpful to review the anatomy since what happens in the systemic circulation may directly affect the cardiopulmonary circulation. Blood enters the heart through the superior and inferior venae cavae and empties into the right atrium. Next it flows through the tricuspid valve into the right ventricle, then through the pulmonary artery to the lungs, where it discards its waste, carbon dioxide (CO_2), and picks up oxygen (O_2). The blood returns through the pulmonary vein to the left atrium of the heart and then flows through the bicuspid valve to the left ventricle. From the left ventricle it enters the aorta, beginning its journey through the systemic circulation.

2. Systemic circulation

This system, especially the peripheral vessels, is used in IV therapy.

a. Direction of circulatory flow. The aorta—the largest vessel—ascends from the left ventricle of the heart. The aorta branches into arteries, which in turn branch into arterioles, or small arteries. The arterioles branch into capillaries, which are thin-walled and permeable for exchange of gases (O_2 for CO_2) and nutrients. Venules—the smallest veins—collect blood from capillaries and deliver it to the veins. Veins bring blood back to the heart's right atrium. To keep blood flowing up toward the heart, veins contain many one-way valves.

b. Pressure. Pressure in veins is lower than in arteries because veins don't have the benefit of the heart's pumping action—hence the need for valves.

c. Elasticity. Arteries have more elastic fibers than do veins. These fibers help the arterial walls to withstand the high pressure of the blood that is pumped through them. As there are fewer elastic fibers in the lining of the veins than in the lining of the arteries, veins can constrict or dilate more readily. A distended vein, because it's less elastic, won't resume its shape as quickly as an artery.

B. STRUCTURE OF ARTERIES AND VEINS

The walls of both arteries and veins consist of three main layers (see Figure 2-1).

1. Tunica intima

a. Composition. This innermost layer consists of endothelium, which is made up of smooth, flat cells. Because it is smooth, blood cells and platelets can flow freely through the lumen. When inserting and removing needles and catheters, be careful not to scratch or roughen this inner surface by unnecessary movement of the device in the vein. Cells and platelets may accumulate in rough places and form a thrombus. The thrombus may eventually block circulation in the vessel or may break off, creating an embolus.

b. Valves. Arteries don't have valves; veins do. Valves are semilunar folds in the endothelial lining. They occur most often in the extremities and at points of branching. Sometimes they cause veins to bulge. Avoid venipuncture just below bulges, as you may otherwise hit and damage a valve.

2. Tunica media

a. Composition. This middle layer consists of muscle, elastic tissue, and nerve fibers. The vasoconstrictors and vasodilators located in this lining permit the veins to contract or dilate in response to various stimuli, such as

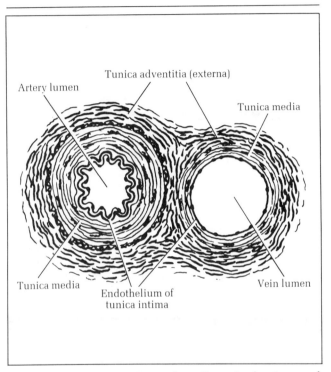

Figure 2-1 Cross sections of medium-sized artery and vein, showing the tunica intima, tunica media, and tunica adventitia (externa) × 250

heat, cold, or drugs. As noted before, this layer is thicker in arteries than in veins.

b. Spasms. Spasms of veins are due to infusion of cold fluids too quickly, to chemical irritation by a drug, to mechanical irritation, or to strong emotional stimuli, such as fear. They can be relieved by applying heat, which dilates the vein and promotes the flow of blood, by calming the patient, or by removing the source of stimulation causing the irritation. Spasm of a vein is less serious than spasm of an artery. Arterial spasm may block circulation, resulting in necrosis and gangrene if not relieved promptly.

3. Tunica adventitia (tunica externa)

a. Composition. This outer layer consists of areolar connective and elastic tissue. It is thicker in arteries than in veins.

b. Function. Its primary function is to hold the vessel together.

C. SUPERFICIAL VEINS OF THE UPPER EXTREMITIES

Each person has a distinctly individual venous network available for peripheral IV infusion. While many of the major veins may be the same, individual variations are expected in peripheral circulation. Figure 2-2 shows the superficial veins of the dorsal aspect of the hand. Peripheral and central veins of the upper body can be seen in Figure 2-3.

1. Digital veins

The dorsal digital veins run along the sides of the fingers and are joined by connecting branches. They can be used when other veins aren't available and will accommodate a small-gauge

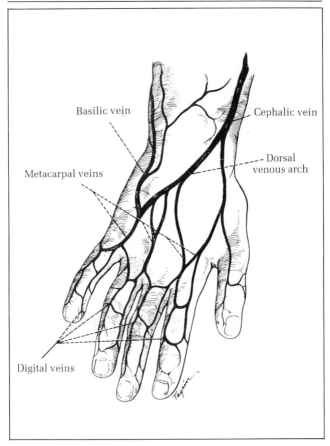

Figure 2-2 Superficial veins of the dorsal aspect of the hand

Reproduced, with permission, from Plumer AL: *Principles and Practice of Intravenous Therapy*, 3rd ed. © 1982, Little, Brown and Company

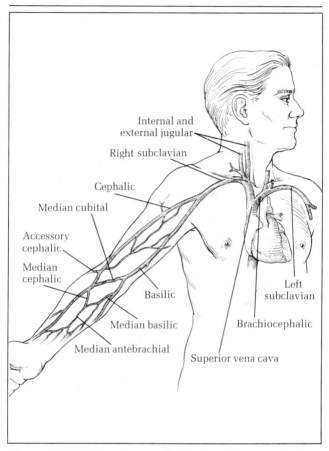

Figure 2-3 Peripheral and central veins of the upper body

winged needle or 22- or 24-gauge CON. When utilizing the digital veins for IV infusions, be sure to tape the device securely in place and properly support it to prevent movement of the joint. A tongue blade may be used as a splint for a specific finger, or a hand board may be applied to support the entire hand.

2. Metacarpal veins

a. Location. These veins are formed by union of the digital veins on the back of the hand and include the metacarpal veins, which make up the dorsal venous arch. They are ideal for IV use: They are usually visible, they lie flat on the back of the hand, and the metacarpal bones act as a splint for the IV device.

b. Venipuncture. In a normal adult, the metacarpal veins are usually the first to be used. Start venipuncture at the most distal point on the extremity. Subsequent venipunctures can then be made above the previous site. This is especially important if the previous site is irritated, phlebotic, or infiltrated.

c. Elderly patients. Take extra care with elderly patients. Their skin and vessels are often very thin and the tissue and muscle support is inadequate. This may make them especially susceptible to fast-forming hematomas.

d. Support. Firm, secure taping is always necessary. In most cases, use a hand board.

3. Cephalic vein

a. Location. The cephalic vein runs upward along the radial border of the forearm, sending branches to both surfaces of the forearm as it goes. It provides an excellent route for IV infusion: It's often visible, it readily accommodates large (low-gauge) catheters/needles, and the radius provides a natural splint.

b. Venipuncture. The cephalic vein may be entered from the wrist area to the upper arm— always using the most distal site first. A hand board is necessary when the IV is located in the wrist area.

4. Accessory cephalic vein

a. Location. The accessory cephalic vein originates from a plexus on the dorsum of the forearm or from the dorsal venous network. It often branches off from the cephalic vein just above the wrist and rejoins it near the elbow. The accessory cephalic readily accepts large catheters/needles and is an excellent choice for transfusions and IV infusions.

b. Venipuncture. The accessory cephalic vein may be entered anywhere along its course, but the most distal site should be used first.

5. Basilic vein

a. Location. The basilic vein originates in the ulnar portion of the dorsal venous network and ascends the ulnar surface of the forearm. Just below the elbow it curves toward the inside of the forearm and meets the median cubital vein. The basilic may be entered anywhere along its course, above as well as below the antecubital fossa.

b. Venipuncture. Because it's inconspicuous, the basilic vein is often overlooked. Always look and feel for it when you're having trouble finding a suitable site. Flex the patient's elbow, so the catheter points in the direction of venous flow, to start the IV infusion.

6. Median antebrachial vein

a. Location. The median antebrachial vein arises from the dorsal venous plexus, runs along the ulnar side of the forearm, and empties into the basilic or median cubital vein. It isn't always easy to find.

b. Venipuncture. The median veins are not generally desirable for IV infusions because they lie near large numbers of nerves, arteries, and other structures. They should be considered as last resorts for infusions into the upper extremities.

7. Median cephalic and median basilic veins

a. Location. These veins are found in the antecubital fossa and are generally used for drawing blood.

b. Infusion. If either of these veins must be used (as a last resort or in an emergency situation), the elbow must be immobilized with a long arm board. This may cause pain and stiffness to the elbow joint. An IV started in this area should be changed as soon as possible to a more suitable location. In case a hematoma begins to develop while initiating an infusion in the antecubital area, don't flex the patient's elbow to attempt to stop the bleeding. Apply digital pressure over the site with a sterile gauze pad and raise the patient's arm until the bleeding stops.

D. ARTERIAL PUNCTURE

Inadvertent puncture of an artery may occur if proper insertion technique is not observed or in two anomalous situations: arteriovenous anastomosis and aberrant arteries.

1. Arteriovenous anastomosis

An arteriovenous anastomosis is a direct opening between an artery and a vein. The vein is therefore filled with high-pressure arterial blood.

> ***a. Causes.*** Anastomosis may be congenital, it may be caused by accidental simultaneous puncture of an adjacent artery and vein, or it may be surgically created (to produce an AV shunt).
>
> ***b. Venipuncture.*** The vein will look unusually large, firm, and tortuous, and will appear to be a good vein. It will pulsate. When it's pierced, the blood may spurt. You'll have difficulty threading a catheter against the force of the blood. Repeated punctures will prove unsuccessful, painful, and injurious to the lining of the vein. If IV tubing is attached, fluids will not flow freely but blood will back up into the tubing toward the solution because of the high pressure of arterial blood.
>
> ***c. What to do.*** Withdraw the catheter/needle, apply pressure over the site with a sterile gauze pad for at least five minutes, and try another site.

2. Aberrant arteries

Aberrant arteries are arteries that are located superficially where they're not expected, or where you may expect to find a vein. They are frequently seen in thin or emaciated persons and often occur bilaterally. Their incidence is approximately 1 in 10 persons.

a. Cause. Aberrant arteries are congenital.

b. Venipuncture. The artery will pulsate. When it's punctured, blood will spurt and will enter a syringe under its own power without aspiration. You'll have difficulty threading a catheter. If you do succeed in threading the catheter, the blood will continue to advance up the tubing. The blood will be bright red, not the darker venous hue.

c. What to do. Withdraw the catheter/needle, apply pressure over the site with a sterile gauze pad for at least five minutes, and try another site. Do not use the same site on the patient's other side, as you may hit the contralateral aberrant artery.

CHAPTER 3

The skin

The skin is important in IV therapy because you must pierce it in order to reach any vein. Familiarity with the skin's thickness and consistency at various venipuncture sites will enable you to pierce it correctly and prevent perforation and infiltration. Proper cleansing of the skin at venipuncture sites (see Chapter 7) is also important, as any organisms present there can enter the patient's circulation via the catheter/needle. The skin consists of two main layers—the epidermis and dermis—and overlies the superficial fascia (see Figure 3-1).

A. EPIDERMIS

The epidermis, or top layer of skin, is composed of horny (squamous) cells that are relatively insensitive. It's the body's first and main line of defense against invasion by microorganisms.

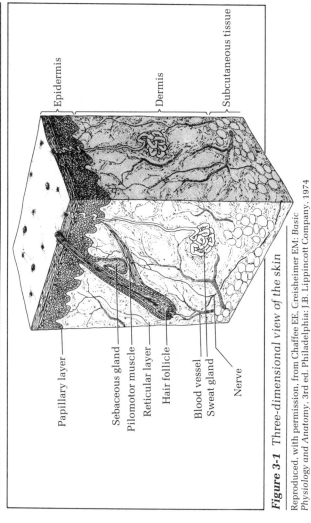

Figure 3-1 Three-dimensional view of the skin

Reproduced, with permission, from Chaffee EE, Greisheimer EM: *Basic Physiology and Anatomy*, 3rd ed. Philadelphia: J.B. Lippincott Company, 1974

1. Thickness
The epidermis is thickest on the palms of the hands and soles of the feet and thinnest on the inner surfaces of the extremities. Thickness also varies with age and physical condition.

2. Catheter/needle insertion
The angle of insertion will be more perpendicular to the skin where the epidermis is thicker, and closer to the skin where the epidermis is thinner.

B. DERMIS

The dermis lies directly under, and is much thicker than, the epidermis. The dermis houses blood vessels, hair follicles, sweat and sebaceous glands, small muscles, and nerves.

1. Thickness
The thickness of the dermis varies on different parts of the body and is also dependent on age and physical condition.

2. Sensitivity
Because the skin is an organ of touch, it contains many small blood vessels and afferent nerves and is highly sensitive. It reacts quickly to temperature, touch, pressure, and painful stimuli. The number of nerve fibers varies in different parts of the body, so that some areas are more sensitive than others.

3. Catheter/needle insertion
Most of the pain associated with starting an IV infusion occurs in the heavily innervated, highly vascular dermis. Therefore, insert your catheter/needle through these two layers as quickly and smoothly as possible.

C. SUPERFICIAL FASCIA

The superficial fascia consists of subcutaneous fibroareolar connective tissue. It lies below the epidermis and dermis, provides a covering for the blood vessels, and varies in thickness. It is found over almost the entire surface of the body connecting the skin with the deep or aponeurotic fascia. As infection in the tissue of the superficial fascia spreads easily throughout the body, it is very important to use careful aseptic technique for insertion and maintenance of IV devices.

CHAPTER 4

Shock

When starting an IV line in an emergency, remember that most traumatically injured people are in some sort of shock.

A. DEFINITION OF SHOCK

Shock occurs when the pumping action of the heart is insufficient in maintaining the flow of blood through the vessels. As a result, the peripheral vessels constrict and the circulatory pattern shifts in order to sustain the supply of oxygenated blood to vital organs, especially the heart, lungs, kidneys, and brain. The degree of constriction depends on the degree and type of shock.

B. TYPES OF SHOCK

The list below contains only some of the many different types of shock.

▶ Hypovolemic—due to loss of fluid through hemorrhage (internal or external), burns, vomiting, diarrhea, or severe hyperglycemia in diabetics
▶ Neurogenic—due to peripheral vascular dilation as a result of nerve stimulation or nerve block, as in spinal cord injuries
▶ Cardiogenic—due to failure of the heart to pump sufficient blood
▶ Respiratory—due to lack of inspired oxygen, as in narcotic overdoses or drug-alcohol interactions
▶ Septic (or toxic)—due to widespread infection or poisoning
▶ Psychogenic—due to overwhelming emotion, such as fright (including fear of injection)
▶ Anaphylactic—due to allergy to a drug or foreign protein.

C. RECOGNITION OF SHOCK

Constriction of the peripheral vessels produces several characteristic signs:

▶ Pallor of skin, lips, eyelids, gums, tongue
▶ Cool, moist skin, often beaded with cold sweat
▶ Rapid breathing
▶ Hypotension and widening pulse pressure
▶ Weak, rapid, thready pulse
▶ Anxiety, clouded senses, disorientation
▶ Low urinary output and/or thirst.

D. TREATMENT

Treatment of shock is based on several principles, but it must be prompt and appropriate to the cause and degree of shock.

1. Open airway
Maintain an open airway and support respiration.
Failure to keep the airway open is the most
common cause of death in shock patients.

2. Stop hemorrhage
Locate accessible external hemorrhage sites.
Apply compression dressings to reduce fluid loss.

3. Cardiopulmonary resuscitation
Preserve normal cardiac and respiratory function
by applying CPR as needed.

4. Volume replacement

a. IV fluids. These include lactated Ringer's
solution, saline, dextrose, serum albumin,
plasma protein fraction, dextran, packed red
cells, and fresh frozen red cells; whole blood
is now rarely used. Chapter 13 discusses
these fluid preparations and their
compatibility in more detail.

b. Trendelenburg position. Raising the
lower extremities increases the blood supply
to the heart, lungs, kidneys, and brain.
However, because this position pushes the
abdominal viscera up against the diaphragm,
reducing the patient's breathing capacity,
some now recommend elevating only the
patient's feet.

c. Inflatable antishock trousers. These
appliances, by constricting the legs and lower
abdomen, increase the blood supply to vital
organs. They should only be applied, or
removed, by personnel specifically trained
in their proper use.

E. SEVERITY AND COMPLICATIONS

1. Slight degree of shock

a. An average deficit of 1 liter of blood or a blood pressure 20% below normal.

b. It is reversible.

2. Moderate degree of shock

a. An average deficit of 1.8 liters of blood or a blood pressure 35% below normal.

b. It is also reversible if treated promptly.

3. Severe degree of shock

a. An average deficit of 2.5 liters of blood or a blood pressure 50% below normal.

b. It is an acute condition that may progress rapidly to irreversibility and death.

4. Disseminated intravascular coagulation

a. Definition. Disseminated intravascular coagulation (DIC) is a clinical condition manifested by an imbalance in the body's blood coagulation system. It is the result of an underlying disease process. Blood begins to clot within the peripheral circulation, followed by excessive, diffuse fibrinolysis.

b. Cause. DIC may be activated by injury to the body's tissues, red blood cells, or endothelial cells. Some common events that may precipitate the DIC process include heat stroke, near drowning, cardiac arrest, septicemia, extensive burns, major chest trauma or surgery, hemorrhage, cancer of the lung or prostate, leukemia, obstetrical accidents, chemotherapy, snake bites, and major organ failure.

c. Recognition and treatment. DIC may vary from obscure internal bleeding to mild oozing from the skin, GI tract, GU tract, or wound, to profuse hemorrhaging. It may begin insidiously or suddenly. Blood loss should be carefully measured and blood replacement should be an integral part of the therapy. Treatment should be aimed at alleviating the underlying cause and should be supported by use of appropriate drugs and intravenous fluids. It is vitally important that DIC be recognized rapidly and treatment initiated promptly if serious consequences, including possible death, are to be prevented.

F. THE PATIENT IN SHOCK

Always treat shock seriously. It can progress rapidly from a slight state to one that is irreversible. Remember to treat any life-threatening condition that may be present first, then initiate IV therapy. Intravenous fluids will increase the circulatory volume and help decrease the effects of shock. Don't say anything in front of an unconscious patient that you wouldn't say if the person were conscious. The patient may only appear to be unresponsive. Remember: The sense of hearing is the last to go.

CHAPTER 5

Equipment: ambulance versus hospital

NOTE: Any infusion started in the field should be torn down to the catheter when the patient is admitted to the hospital. Emergency infusions outside the hospital usually are started under less than aseptic conditions. The area should be meticulously cleansed and a new, sterile dressing with antimicrobial ointment or solution applied to minimize the possibility of infection. If the site is grossly contaminated, the IV device should be completely removed as soon as possible and the IV restarted, if necessary, in a new location.

A. BASIC EQUIPMENT

Most ambulances and rescue vehicles need to carry only basic IV equipment. This equipment is practically the same as the basic equipment used in a hospital.

1. IV solution (sterile)

a. Ambulance. Most ambulances carry only three kinds of IV solutions:

- 500 ml of 5% dextrose in water (D_5W)—for medical emergencies
- Liter (1,000 ml) of lactated Ringer's solution (R/L)—for traumatic emergencies
- Liter (1,000 ml) of normal saline (0.9%)—for hypovolemic patients.

b. Hospital. IV solutions are used in the hospital according to the orders of a physician.

c. Containers. IV solutions come in glass bottles, plastic bags, and semirigid plastic bottles.

2. Administration set (sterile)

The standard/straight administration set includes the following parts:

- Spike
- Drip chamber
- Tubing
- Regulator clamp
- Rubber stopper/flash ball or injection ports
- Adapter/connector
- Protective caps.

3. Catheter/needle devices (sterile)

The type of device you use for venipuncture depends on several considerations:

- Purpose of infusion (medication, anesthesia, hydration, nutrition, etc.)
- Size of peripheral vein selected
- Patient's age and condition
- Nature of infusion (continuous, intermittent, one-time bolus).

a. CON. Use the following sizes for stable venous access:

▶ 14- or 16-gauge × 1½ or 2 inches—for multiple major trauma, infusing large amounts of blood or fluid quickly under pressure, and for extensive surgical procedures (transplants, cardiac surgery, etc.)

▶ 18-gauge × 1¼ to 2 inches—for major trauma, major surgery, cardiac arrest, or blood transfusions

▶ 20-gauge × 1¼ to 1½ inches—for minor trauma, minor surgery, blood transfusions when unable to insert an 18-gauge, and for most medical needs

▶ 22-gauge × 1 inch—for routine keep-vein-open (KVO) procedures, pediatric patients (with medical problems), irritating medications; never to be used when any type of surgery is indicated

▶ 24-gauge × ½ or ¾ inch—for infants or when necessary to start an infusion in a digital or scalp vein or a small, spidery vein; never to be used when any type of surgery is indicated.

b. Parts of a CON:

▶ Bevel tip
▶ Needle/stylet
▶ Catheter
▶ Flash chamber
▶ Syringe or vented plug
▶ Hub
▶ Protective cap.

c. Winged needles. Use these sizes for entry into veins for infusions of short duration or when the patient is allergic to the materials used in the CON device:

- ▸ 19-gauge—same as an 18-gauge CON
- ▸ 21-gauge—same as a 20-gauge CON
- ▸ 23-gauge—same as a 22-gauge CON
- ▸ 25-gauge—same as a 24-gauge CON—used for small, spidery veins or for neonates, if you can't insert a CON
- ▸ 27-gauge—smaller than any available CON—used for extremely small veins.

d. Parts of a winged needle:
- ▸ Bevel tip
- ▸ Needle
- ▸ Wings
- ▸ Tubing
- ▸ Adapter (hub)
- ▸ Vented plug
- ▸ Protective cap.

4. Tourniquet

5. Paper, Dermicel, or Transpore tape
NOTE: Do not use adhesive tape. It is extremely hard on a patient's skin.

6. Arm board
- ▸ Short—for the hand or wrist area
- ▸ Long—for IVs located in the antecubital fossa.

7. Dry gauze sponges (2 × 2s or 4 × 4s)

8. Alcohol wipes
NOTE: Because it's often impossible to obtain an allergy history on an emergency patient in the field, ambulances should not carry povidone-iodine products.

9. IV pole or hooks

B. ADDITIONAL EQUIPMENT USED IN A HOSPITAL

1. CTN device

The catheter-through-needle device is used primarily for entering central or deep veins, generally in specialized procedures such as total parenteral nutrition and central venous pressure monitoring. CTN devices are generally inserted in the subclavian, jugular, or brachial veins by a physician or specially trained personnel.

2. Vent

Vents should only be used with unvented glass bottles. Plastic bags and semirigid plastic containers automatically contract as they empty, so the flow rate remains constant without venting.

3. IV tubing with macrodrip chamber

In addition to the basic 10-drop/ml size, standard macrodrip chambers (see Figure 5-1) come in the following sizes:

- ▶ 15 drops/ml
- ▶ 20 drops/ml.

4. IV tubing with microdrip chamber

Microdrip chambers (see Figure 5-2) deliver 60 drops/ml and are used for various purposes:

- ▶ To deliver small amounts of medication over long periods
- ▶ To regulate the flow of medication very precisely
- ▶ To keep a vein open.

5. Filter

Filters come in various pore sizes:

- ▶ 1 to 5 μm—removes particles but not bacteria

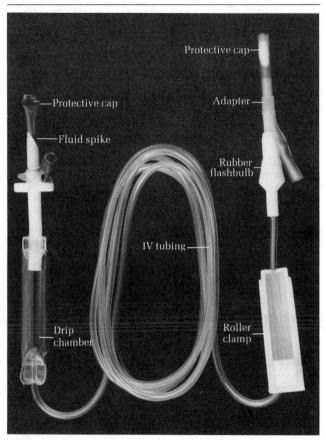

Figure 5-1 Macrodrip tubing

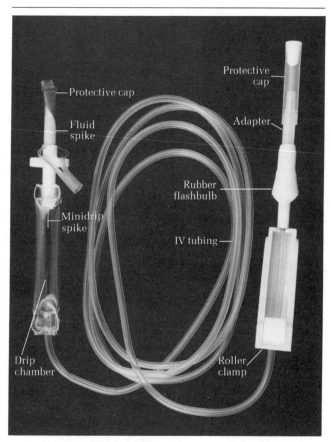

Figure 5-2 Microdrip tubing

▶ 0.45 μm—removes most bacteria and particulate matter

▶ 0.22 μm—removes all bacteria, fungi, yeasts, and particulate matter.

6. Gravity-feed piggyback set

A piggyback is a secondary set used for intermittent drug administration. It runs into the upper Y port of the primary IV line. Because the piggyback bottle must hang higher than the primary bottle, in order for the infusion to run by gravity, an extension hook for the primary bottle is provided.

7. Simultaneous infusion

A second IV tubing may be attached to the lower Y port of the primary line for simultaneous infusion of a second fluid. Both containers of fluid may hang at the same height.

8. Volume-control chamber

A volume-control set, or fluid chamber, is used to deliver small amounts of medication diluted in precise quantities of fluid. It may be used as the primary set for an infant or small child, or for an adult requiring precise measurements of fluids and/or medications. Because a volume-control chamber is easily contaminated (by frequent injections into the system), a piggyback setup is generally preferred whenever possible.

9. Stopcock

A stopcock (Figure 5-3) may be added to an IV line to provide for direct injection of a medication.

NOTE: Whenever a stopcock is added to an IV line, extra care must be taken to ensure that the ports remain covered and that the entire infusion system doesn't become contaminated.

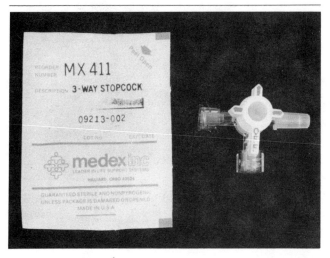

Figure 5-3 *Stopcock*

10. Dressings
The following types of dressings may be used:

- Sterile gauze pad (2 × 2)
- Band-Aid (sterile)
- Transparent film (sterile).

11. Blood transfusion sets
There are several types of transfusion sets:

- Straight-line set with built-in blood filter—for whole blood, packed red cells, frozen cells, or washed cells
- Y set—when saline is needed, as with packed red cells or whole blood through a secondary line
- Microaggregate filter set—for large amounts (more than three units) of packed red cells,

frozen cells, or washed cells; also for immunosuppressed patients or those with potential febrile leukocyte reactions
▸ Component syringe set—for platelets or cryoprecipitates when infusing by IV push
▸ Component drip set—for platelets or cryoprecipitates when infusing by IV drip.

When large quantities of blood must be administered quickly, extra equipment is needed:

▸ Transfusion pump—either built-in or slip-on
▸ Blood-warming device—immersible coil or electric warmer.

12. Intermittent-infusion reservoir (PRN adapter)

There are four main types of reservoirs that are used to keep a vein open but that allow a patient mobility:

▸ Standard heparin lock (winged infusion device)
▸ Adapter plug used with standard needle
▸ Adapter plug with flexible CON (Figure 5-4)
▸ Latex seal attached to CON device.

13. Infusion pumps and controllers

Various types of pumps and controllers are available and serve a variety of needs:

▸ Syringe pumps—used for very slow and precise infusions and KVO rates (0.01 ml/hour)
▸ Peristaltic pumps—move fluid through the tubing with a peristaltic, wavelike motion (most peristaltic pumps will deliver 1 to 300 ml/hour)
▸ Piston-action (volumetric) pumps—the most versatile (deliver 1 to 999 ml/hour)
▸ Controllers—work by gravity flow. Controllers vary in their delivery ranges (most deliver 1 to 300 ml/hour).

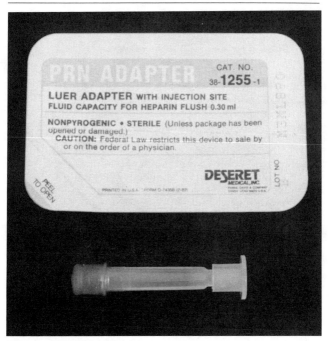

Figure 5-4 PRN adapter

14. Special additional equipment for central lines
▶ Occlusive tape or transparent dressing
▶ Radiopaque CTN catheter (8 to 12 inches).

15. Swabs or wipes
▶ Alcohol and acetone
▶ Povidone-iodine
▶ Skin protector (tincture of benzoin, skin guard).

16. Povidone-iodine ointment

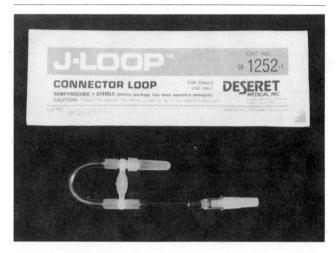

Figure 5-5 IV loop

17. IV stand

18. Obturator
An obturator fits inside the catheter and acts as a plug. The obturator will keep the catheter patent, while the tubing is disconnected, without the need to inject a heparinized solution.

19. IV loop
An IV loop (Figure 5-5) may be attached to the end of the catheter/needle device to replace the loop made with the IV tubing. This helps prevent kinking of the tubing and facilitates tubing changes.

CHAPTER 6

Preparing IV equipment

Whether you're starting an infusion in the hospital or in the field, always assemble and inspect all your equipment before you touch the patient. Maintain sterile technique.

A. HAND WASHING

Wash your hands vigorously with antimicrobial soap before beginning the procedure and before going on to each subsequent patient, whether you're starting an IV line or merely changing bottles, bags, tubing, or dressings, injecting medications into a line, or disconnecting a line.

B. INSPECTING YOUR EQUIPMENT

1. IV solution
Check the bottle or bag carefully for:

► Cracks, leaks, tightness of seals
► Cloudiness, discoloration, precipitation

▸ Correctness of solution
▸ Expiration date.

If a solution has turned cloudy, consider it contaminated and don't use it.

2. Catheter/needle

> *a. Catheter.* Discard the device if the catheter is bumpy or torn at the ends.
>
> *b. Needle.* Does the bevel look perfectly sharp and the shaft perfectly smooth?
>
> *c. Hub.* Does it lock tightly?
>
> *d. Size.* Is the size appropriate for the purpose of the infusion?

3. Tubing

> *a. Size and type.* Make sure the tubing is the right length and has the necessary ports, clamps, filters, and other devices.
>
> *b. Leaks.* As you prime the tubing by running fluid through it to remove air (see section C5 below), check for leaks, especially around ports and connections.

4. Other devices

Carry out a thorough inspection of each extra device you'll be adding to the line.

C. SPIKING AND PRIMING

1. Flow clamp

Slide the clamp up the tubing until it's just below the drip chamber. Close the clamp.

> *a. Roller clamp.* To adjust the rate of flow to the desired flow rate, the roller is rolled up to open the line and down to close the line.
>
> *b. Screw clamp.* To adjust the rate of flow to the desired flow rate, the screw is turned

clockwise to close the line and counterclockwise to open the line.

c. Slide clamp. When using a slide clamp, the rate of flow cannot be adjusted, only turned on or off. To close the line, the tubing is slid into the narrow end of the clamp; to open the line, the tubing is slid to the wide end of the clamp.

2. Spiking

a. Nonvented bottle. Remove the cap and wipe the rubber stopper with alcohol. Remove the cover from a vented spike and push the spike firmly into the stopper.

b. Vented bottle. Remove the cap and latex cover. If you don't hear a hiss, the bottle's vacuum has been breached and the solution is contaminated. Discard it. If you hear a hiss, remove the cover from a nonvented spike and insert the spike into the larger of the two holes, after wiping the stopper with alcohol.

c. Plastic bags. If the bag is the kind with a large port and broad lip, it need not be hung before spiking. The other kind must be hung first. Remove the protective caps from the bag and the tubing spike, and insert the spike into the bag with a twisting motion.

3. Hanging

Hang bottles and bags so that all vents and secondary ports face outward. Hang all solutions a distance of at least 40 to 45 inches higher than the venipuncture site.

4. Drip chamber

Gently squeeze the drip chamber until it's about half full of solution. This will help prevent air bubbles from forming in the tubing.

5. Priming the tubing

The purpose of priming, or flushing, the tubing is to remove air and any particulate matter from the line. The average tubing contains between 5 and 15 ml of air.

a. Vented cap. If the tubing has a vented protective cap, prime the tubing by opening the clamp and filling the tubing with solution. Gently tap at any air bubbles. Invert any secondary ports or valves and tap at them to release air bubbles. When the tubing is full and no air bubbles remain, close the clamp.

b. Nonvented cap. If the cap isn't vented, you must remove it to flush the air out. Protect the cap from contamination. Hold the end of the tubing over a sink or wastebasket, open the clamp, and let the solution run through. Tap away all air bubbles as described above. When no bubbles remain, close the clamp. Replace the cap or cover the end with a sterile needle and cap.

6. Hanging the tubing

Loop the primed tubing over the top of the IV pole to keep it safe while you prep the patient and perform venipuncture. Be careful to maintain the sterility of the connector (end of the tubing) by keeping it capped until you are ready to connect it to the patient's infusion system.

CHAPTER **7**

Preparing the patient for IV therapy

A. APPROACHING THE PATIENT

1. Identification
Address the patient by name, and also check the ID band to make sure you are about to treat the right person.

2. Reassurance
Introduce yourself politely and tell the patient what you're going to do. Ask the patient's cooperation in holding still while you perform venipuncture. As you work, continue to give the patient overt and covert reassurance. Emotional tension may cause venous spasms and make venipuncture more difficult.

3. Allergies
Unless you're working under emergency conditions, you should check the patient's chart for

a history of allergies. Find out whether the patient is allergic to:

- ▶ Medications, or items in the solution you're about to infuse
- ▶ Iodine
- ▶ Tape.

4. Clotting disorders and other conditions
Find out whether the patient has a clotting problem or has been taking any medication that might be incompatible with the one you're about to give. If the patient is about to have a mastectomy or nephrectomy, or surgery on an arm or hip, make sure you know which side.

B. SELECTING A VEIN

In selecting a vein for venipuncture, consider the size, condition, and location of veins, the patient's age, size, and clinical status, special tests or procedures the patient is undergoing, and the purpose and type of the IV procedure.

1. Size of the vein
Larger peripheral veins are easier to find and enter than smaller veins, and they pose less risk of perforation and infiltration or extravasation.

> *a. Shock.* A patient in severe shock may have collapsed veins, making it all the more difficult to find a vein for venipuncture.

> *b. Drugs.* Veins may be widened or narrowed by drugs with vasodilating or vasoconstricting properties, respectively.

2. Condition of the vein
> *a. Palpation.* Always palpate the extremity before you choose a vein. Often the more visible veins aren't as suitable for IV infusion

as deeper veins that can only be palpated. Palpate for resiliency and also to make sure that you do indeed have a vein and not an artery, aberrant artery, or arteriovenous anastomosis (see Chapter 2).

b. Phlebotic or infiltrated area. If a vein is phlebotic or the area infiltrated due to a previous IV, restart the IV in the opposite limb if at all possible. If the same limb needs to be used, you must restart the infusion *above* the phlebotic or infiltrated area to avoid any further trauma or irritation to the veins and/or tissues at the affected site.

c. Veins to avoid. Avoid veins that are:

- Tortuous
- Hardened or scarred from age or previous IV use
- Sore or inflamed from recent use
- Filled with bifurcations or large, prominent valves.

3. Location of the vein

Chapter 2 outlines the anatomy of the peripheral venous circulation in detail, but locations for venipuncture are listed here for quick review.

a. Upper extremities. Remember that the force of gravity aids venous return to the heart, and that you should always start venipuncture at the most distal site possible. Therefore, the best veins are those of the upper extremities, starting with the hands. From best to worst:

- Back of the hand
- Wrist
- Outer aspect of the forearm
- Inner aspect of the forearm

▶ Upper arm
▶ Antecubital fossa.

Use the antecubital fossa only when no other peripheral veins are available in the upper extremities. In fact, some authorities completely reject the antecubital fossa for catheter insertion—although it's ideal for giving injections and drawing blood samples. For infusion, it's necessary to immobilize the elbow joint with a long arm board to prevent extravasation, kinking of the catheter, or damage to underlying arteries and nerves. Prolonged immobilization causes painful stiffness. An IV infusion started in the antecubital fossa should be moved at the earliest opportunity.

b. Other parts of the body. The jugular, subclavian, and other deep veins are ordinarily reserved for special procedures such as total parenteral nutrition. Except in infants, in whom a scalp vein is usually preferable, the following are the locations of last resort:

▶ Scalp
▶ Feet, ankles, and legs.

Depending on institutional policy, a physician's order may be necessary to start an infusion in a lower extremity.

c. Side of the body. Certain surgical procedures may necessitate that the IV be placed on a specific side:

▶ Patients having surgery on an arm or a breast will generally have the IV started on the opposite limb

▸ Patients having surgery on a hip, kidney, or lung may generally have the IV started on the surgical side
▸ For further clarification or specific instructions concerning which side may be best for starting the IV, you may want to check with the patient's physician or anesthesiologist
▸ For medical patients, use the side opposite the hand the patient normally prefers, if possible.

4. Age of the patient

a. Infants. To simplify problems of restraint, a scalp vein is usually preferred. When using a scalp vein, point the bevel of the needle toward the patient's face.

b. Geriatric patients. Veins in elderly patients may be hardened, or fragile and easily torn. They're also likely to be made tortuous by sluggish circulation.

5. Size of the patient

a. Obese patients. The veins of the hand, wrist, or inner forearm may be seen after you've used a tourniquet, but they may be difficult to palpate. You may have to increase the angle of insertion of the catheter/needle in order to penetrate the extra adipose tissue.

b. Thin or emaciated patients. In especially thin patients, you're likely to see fragile, "rolling" veins under thin, papery skin. You'll need to anchor the vein very firmly, lower the angle of insertion of the catheter/needle, and use the direct approach for venipuncture (see Chapter 8).

6. Clinical status of the patient

a. Injured extremity. Never start an IV on an injured or diseased extremity, on the stump of an amputated limb, or on an extremity where the pulse is weak or absent.

b. Position of patient. If the patient must lie prone or on one side, your choice of vein is limited to the exposed aspect of his/her body.

c. Mastectomy. Start an IV on the side opposite the mastectomy. If the patient has had bilateral mastectomies, start the IV in the arm with less edema. Such a patient must be watched closely for increased edema and signs of sepsis.

d. Arteriovenous fistula or shunt. Start IVs on the opposite arm. If you must use the same arm as the one with the shunt, use the upper arm, never the forearm or the hand. Do not leave the tourniquet on the shunt arm for more than one minute; if possible, perform the venipuncture without using a tourniquet. If you do inadvertently puncture an AV fistula, remove the catheter/needle, elevate the patient's arm, and apply pressure to the site for 10 minutes. Notify the physician. When starting an IV in a scalp vein of an infant with an AV shunt, perform venipuncture on the side of the head opposite the shunt. Don't leave the rubber band on the patient's head any longer than necessary, and don't place it directly over the shunt.

e. Mental state. Even if a patient is unconscious when you start an IV, you must consider the possibility that he/she may wake up confused and agitated. If this seems likely, restraints should probably be used according to your institution's policy. It may also be necessary to restrain a child who is too young to cooperate.

7. Special tests and procedures

a. Angiograms, arteriograms, and aortograms. Check the patient's chart to see which side is being prepped, and start the IV on the opposite side. Since most such patients have cardiac and/or circulatory problems, fluid overload is especially dangerous. Make sure the patient's nurse knows an IV has been started so that she can watch the patient closely for signs of circulatory overload.

b. Pacemaker insertion (transvenous). Always start the IV in the arm opposite the pacemaker site. If the IV is in the same arm as the pacemaker catheter, it's difficult to watch for infiltration, as the arm is completely wrapped during catheter insertion. You may consult the physician or radiologist as to his/her preference for the left or right side.

c. Pancreatic duct cannulation. Always start the infusion according to the physician's or radiologist's specifications.

8. Purpose and type of IV procedure

a. Irritating substances. If the patient is to receive hypertonic fluids or drugs that are irritating, the size of the vein is extremely important. In general, the larger the vein in relation to the catheter/needle, the greater the dilution of fluid being administered and the less irritating the infusion. Also, there's less chance that a small-caliber catheter/needle will come in continuous contact with the opposite wall of the vein, and this helps minimize irritation. When it's necessary to infuse highly concentrated or highly irritating solutions, it may be necessary to use central veins such as the subclavian or external jugular.

b. Prolonged administration. If you know that the IV will be in place for several days, it's especially important to choose a site that affords the patient as much comfort and mobility as possible. If you still must place the IV in a movable area such as the hand or wrist, use a short hand board or long arm board. This will help keep irritation to a minimum, decrease the possibility of infiltration, and prevent damage to underlying arteries or nerves.

c. Intermittent-infusion reservoirs, transfusions, and total parenteral nutrition (TPN). These special IV procedures are covered in Chapters 12, 16, and 18, respectively.

C. PREPARING THE SITE

1. Filling the vein
It isn't always necessary to use a tourniquet. If the patient has a high blood pressure or if the veins are large and/or tortuous, you may not need to apply a tourniquet.

2. Distending the vein
a. Gravity. Have the patient hold the extremity lower than the heart. This will slow venous return and fill the distal portion of the vein with blood.

b. Milking. Milk the patient's arm from the proximal to the distal end. This will move blood mechanically down toward the hand.

c. Tourniquet. Apply the tourniquet 3 to 4 inches above the anticipated puncture site, without pinching the skin or pulling hair. You can improvise a tourniquet from such items as these:

- ▶ Soft rubber tubing tied with a slipknot
- ▶ A blood-pressure cuff inflated to slightly above diastolic pressure
- ▶ A Velcro strap.

In field emergencies, it's possible to use a rope, necktie, belt, or scarf. Don't make the tourniquet so tight that it restricts arterial flow. You can check this by feeling for a radial pulse after applying the tourniquet.

d. Tapping. Lightly tapping the puncture area after applying the tourniquet will help distend the vein.

e. Fist clenching. Alternate clenching and relaxation of the patient's fist will help distend the veins. However, if the IV is to be started in the hand, it's best that the hand be relaxed during insertion of the device.

f. Releasing the tourniquet. If venous fill seems insufficient, you may briefly release the tourniquet and then retie it to trap additional venous blood in the extremity.

g. Compresses. Wrap the entire limb in a moist Turkish towel heated to a maximum temperature of 105°F. Cover it with a water-repellent wrapping and leave it in place for 15 to 20 minutes.

h. Sclerosed veins. Sclerosed veins require very little pressure from a tourniquet. In fact, venipuncture may be easier without a tourniquet if the veins are engorged with high-pressure blood.

NOTE: Sclerosed veins may feel hard when palpated. They are *not* a good choice for venipuncture because the lumen of the vein has been narrowed and it may be difficult to enter the vein successfully.

i. Relaxation. A very tense patient may develop spasms or constriction of the veins. Reassurance is very important.

3. Cleansing the site

If the area around the venipuncture site is exceptionally dirty, cleanse it with soap and water or 70% isopropyl alcohol before proceeding to one of the following methods.

a. Povidone-iodine. Using a firm, circular motion from the center to the periphery of an area about 2 inches in diameter, wipe the anticipated puncture site and allow the solution to remain on the skin for at least two minutes. Do not wipe it off. If the povidone-iodine solution is allowed to remain on the skin, its bactericidal effect will continue functioning under the IV dressing.

b. Tincture of iodine. An alternative to povidone-iodine is 2% tincture of iodine in 70% alcohol. Apply the solution as you would the povidone-iodine, allow it to dry for 30 to 60 seconds, and wipe it off with 70% alcohol. Lightly wipe the puncture site—not the entire area—with a sterile gauze pad in order to minimize irritation from the alcohol at the puncture site.

c. Alcohol. If the patient is allergic to iodine, or if no iodine is available, you may cleanse the area with 70% isopropyl alcohol for a minimum of one full minute, using at least three different alcohol wipes. Use a firm, circular, center-to-periphery motion. Allow 30 to 60 seconds for drying, or lightly wipe the puncture site with a sterile gauze pad.

4. Shaving

There is no good evidence for shaving. On the contrary, shaving may be harmful because it produces microabrasions that can harbor bacteria. The antiseptic used to cleanse skin is equally effective on hair. However, if the hair around the site is excessively thick, you may:

▸ Clip it with scissors
▸ Back the tape, or place a gauze pad under the tape when securing the catheter in place (see Chapter 9).

CHAPTER 8

<hr>

Venipuncture technique

<hr>

A. INSERTION

Maintain sterile technique at all times. Never use a catheter/needle for more than one venipuncture; use a new setup and complete prep for each new puncture.

1. Anchoring the vein

With your left hand (if right-handed), hold the patient's arm and stretch the skin with your left thumb. This stretching tension is important to anchor the vein and keep it from rolling while you insert the catheter/needle. If the vein does start to roll, use firmer tension. Pulling the skin taut will enable the needle to pierce the skin more easily, allowing a nontraumatic entrance into the vein and less pain for the patient. Make sure your left thumb is out of the way of the catheter/needle; if you touch the catheter/needle, it is contaminated and must be discarded.

2. Holding the catheter/needle

a. CON. Grasp the catheter by the clear plastic flash chamber, or syringe, behind the hub. Don't grasp the hub itself; if you do, the catheter may slide down over the bevel of the stylet, damaging the catheter, the patient's skin, and the vein.

b. Winged needles. Grasp the wings. Do not touch the needle itself; if you do, it is contaminated and must be discarded. You may wish to connect the winged-needle device to the IV tubing and flush the needle with solution prior to sticking the patient.

c. CTN. Grasp the protective sleeve behind the needle hub.

3. Placing the catheter/needle

Point the device, bevel up, in the direction of venous flow.

a. Indirect method. Place the bevel about $1/4$ inch below, and to the side of, the point where you plan to enter the vein. This method is useful for patients with tough skin.

b. Direct method. Place the bevel directly over the point of venipuncture. This is a useful method for patients with fragile or rolling veins.

4. Piercing the skin

Hold the catheter/needle at a 15° to 45° angle, depending on the texture of the patient's skin (use a sharper angle for tougher skin). Always warn the patient that you're about to insert a needle, to prevent jumping or flinching in surprise. Then push the catheter/needle into the skin, quickly and with a firm, steady motion.

5. Entering the vein

After piercing the skin, immediately lower the catheter/needle until it's almost parallel to the skin. Aim directly for the vein. You may sometimes feel a snap or pop when you enter the vein.

When blood appears in the flash chamber of the CON or the tubing of the winged-needle device, lower the needle even more and slowly continue to advance the catheter/needle another $1/4$ to $1/2$ inch. Now, if a syringe is attached to the device, aspirate to verify good blood return. If you are using a winged needle, finish threading the needle up the vein, release the tourniquet and skin tension, connect the tubing, and start the infusion.

6. Threading the catheter

   a. CON. Either of the following techniques can be used:

   ▶ One-hand technique: While maintaining tension on the skin with one hand, grasp the hub of the catheter and disengage the catheter from the needle or stylet $1/4$ to $1/2$ inch, with the same hand used to perform the venipuncture. Disengaging the catheter will prevent accidental piercing of the vein with the needle while threading the catheter. Holding the hub of the catheter, advance the catheter up the vein and into position. Immediately place a sterile gauze pad or alcohol wipe under the hub of the catheter. Aspirate once again if the device has a syringe attached. Once you are assured that you have good blood return, verifying that you are still within the vein, release the tourniquet and tension on the patient's skin.

▶ Two-hand technique: Once you have entered the vein, verified by a flashback of blood, advance the catheter an additional $\frac{1}{4}$ to $\frac{1}{2}$ inch. Release the skin tension and use that hand to grasp the hub of the catheter and disengage the catheter from the stylet/needle. Holding the stylet/needle securely with one hand, thread the catheter up the vein and into position with the other hand. Aspirate once again if the device has a syringe attached. Once you are assured that you have good blood return, verifying that you are still within the vein, release the tourniquet.

NOTE: Both techniques are acceptable. However, the one-hand technique generally realizes a greater percentage of success, especially for the inexperienced. Retraction of the patient's skin when released may be great enough for the vein to draw back off the catheter/needle, causing it to come out of the vein and resulting in an unsuccessful venipuncture.

b. CTN. Place the flow-control plug in the female adapter. With your left hand, grasp the hub to stabilize the needle. With your right hand, grasp the catheter through the protective sleeve and gently push it into the vein. Remove your left hand from the hub, and grasp the catheter with your left thumb and forefinger to hold it in place as you continue to push with your right hand. As soon as the catheter is fully advanced into the vein, release the tourniquet.

NOTE: As various types of CTN devices are now available, the manufacturer's instructions should be followed to ensure the proper insertion technique for the particular device.

c. Resistance. If you encounter resistance when threading a catheter (either a CON or a CTN), try loosening the tourniquet. If that doesn't help, try this procedure:

- Release the tourniquet
- Disengage and remove the stylet
- If there is good blood return, attach the primed IV tubing to the catheter
- Open the clamp and allow the IV solution to flow into the vein
- If no swelling appears and the fluid seems to be flowing, gently try to float the catheter up the vein and into position.

Under no circumstances should you reinsert the needle or stylet into the catheter once it has been removed.

7. Removing the stylet

a. CON. Pull back on the needle and press lightly on the catheter tip with a finger. You must see some evidence of blood return. If no blood appears on the gauze pad or alcohol wipe, do not connect the IV tubing. The catheter may have become dislodged or perforated the vein. Aspirate again. If you can't aspirate any blood, withdraw the catheter, discard it, and start over at a new site. If you do see evidence of blood return, you're ready to connect the IV tubing.

b. CTN. Gently apply pressure over the vein, using a sterile gauze pad, and withdraw the needle. Maintain pressure for one minute. Then slip the needle protector under the needle so that the needle is in the middle and a portion of the catheter is also enclosed. Snap the needle protector shut. Remove the collar and slide the needle protector back along the catheter until it clicks into the hub. Place a sterile gauze pad under the hub. You are now ready to connect the IV tubing.

NOTE: The technique may vary according to the CTN device being used. Follow the manufacturer's instructions for each device.

B. COMMON DIFFICULTIES WITH VENIPUNCTURE

Repeated unsuccessful attempts to start an infusion may mean that you need to sharpen your venipuncture skills.

1. Not going far enough into the vein

You may not be inserting the needle far enough into the vein. Remember to advance it $\frac{1}{4}$ to $\frac{1}{2}$ inch after you've entered the vein. If you're using a CON, the catheter must be well within the lumen of the vein before you can disengage the stylet and thread the catheter.

2. Tension

You may not be maintaining enough tension on the patient's skin, or maintaining tension long enough. Remember to keep the skin taut during the entire procedure.

3. Angle of entry

You may be inserting the catheter/needle at too steep an angle. You may even be perforating the opposite wall of the vein.

4. Haste

In your desire to spare the patient pain, or to "get it over with" if you're nervous, you may be rushing things. Take your time; it's better for the patient to be stuck only once, the correct way, than to be stuck two or three times.

5. Jabbing

You may be jabbing at the vein instead of smoothly sliding the catheter/needle into it.

6. Approach

You may be using an indirect approach when a direct approach is called for (see section A3 above).

7. When to give up

A common rule of thumb is "Three strikes and you're out." Don't make more than three attempts on the same patient. Get someone else—preferably a person with more experience—to try.

C. USE OF 1% LIDOCAINE LOCAL ANESTHESIA

1. Personnel

Personnel who are permitted to use 1% plain lidocaine (Xylocaine) subcutaneously as a local anesthetic for venipuncture are determined by your institution's policies. They may include:

▶ IV therapists, who are registered nurses
▶ IV technicians, who are specially trained paraprofessionals
▶ Properly trained registered nurses
▶ Physicians.

2. When to use local anesthesia

▶ Routinely for insertion of a catheter larger than 18 gauge in a conscious patient
▶ For any patient—especially a child—who is very apprehensive
▶ For any patient who requests it
▶ Upon a physician's request.

Never use lidocaine for patients who are allergic to it or related local anesthetics (e.g., bupivacaine, Marcaine; etidocaine, Duranest; and mepivacaine, Carbocaine).

3. Procedure

- Wipe the stopper of the vial with alcohol
- Attach a 25-gauge, $\frac{5}{8}$-inch needle to a sterile syringe, or use a tuberculin syringe
- Draw up 1 to 1.5 ml of 1% plain lidocaine using aseptic technique, and expel all air
- Apply a tourniquet, select the site for venipuncture, and remove the tourniquet
- Thoroughly cleanse the area around the site with 70% isopropyl alcohol
- Wipe the area with a sterile gauze pad to remove the alcohol
- Insert the tip of the needle into the subcutaneous tissue at a 15° to 30° angle
- Aspirate; if no blood appears, inject a small amount of lidocaine to produce a small wheal
- Advance the needle and aspirate again; if no blood appears, inject some more lidocaine to produce a small wheal
- After injecting the lidocaine, withdraw the needle and gently rub the injection site with a sterile gauze pad
- Perform venipuncture.

If you aspirate blood, don't inject any lidocaine. Instead, withdraw the needle, gently apply pressure to the site with a sterile gauze pad, and start over at a new site. Don't inject more than 1.5 ml of lidocaine at any time, and always use *plain* lidocaine.

CHAPTER **9**

Starting an IV infusion

A. CONNECTING THE TUBING

1. Adapter
Remove the protective cap from the end of the tubing and connect the tubing to the hub on the venipuncture set.

2. Checking the flow
Open the clamp to make sure the IV solution will flow freely.

3. Checking for infiltration
If the area around the venipuncture site becomes swollen or painful after the solution has begun to enter the vein, the solution may be infiltrating the surrounding tissue. If so:

- Close the clamp
- Withdraw the catheter/needle
- Apply pressure to the site with a sterile gauze pad until the bleeding stops. Cover the site with a sterile Band-Aid

► Pick a new site and begin the procedure again
► Apply warm, moist compresses to the infiltrated area to speed up absorption of the IV solution in the surrounding tissue.

4. Clamping the tubing

Set the regulator clamp at a slow (KVO) rate while you do the next two steps, cleansing and taping.

B. CLEANSING THE VENIPUNCTURE SITE

1. Blood

With a sterile gauze pad, wipe the area clean of any blood. Blood is an excellent medium for bacterial growth and must not be left around the puncture site.

2. Antimicrobial ointment

Cover the venipuncture site with a small amount of povidone-iodine ointment unless you're outside the hospital setting or the patient is sensitive to iodine. It's important to use a preparation that's antifungal as well as antibacterial. Povidone-iodine is effective in killing gram-positive and gram-negative bacteria, including antibiotic-resistant strains, fungi, viruses, protozoa, and yeasts. Use of an ointment that has only antibacterial properties will encourage overgrowth of fungi and antibiotic-resistant strains of bacteria in the warm, moist environment under the IV dressing. Povidone-iodine solution left on the patient's skin during the prepping procedure is also acceptable as a protective agent in place of the ointment.

C. TAPING THE IV DEVICE

All IV devices must be securely taped to the patient's skin. This helps prevent catheter or needle embolism, perforation, dislodgement, and trauma to the inside of the vein. Movement of the catheter/needle inside the vein is not only irritating but also enlarges the percutaneous opening so that bacteria can enter. NOTE: Tape is not sterile. Never cover the venipuncture site directly with tape; use a sterile gauze pad, Band-Aid, or transparent dressing.

1. Looping the tubing

Always loop the tubing and firmly tape the loop to the patient's skin. This helps to stabilize the catheter/needle and also brings the tubing back out of the way of the patient, attendant personnel, and visitors. IV loop devices may be attached to the end of the IV tubing to form this loop.

2. Chevron method

The chevron method of taping (Figure 9-1) may be used with winged needles, CONs, and CTNs.

- Slip a piece of ½-inch tape, sticky side up, under the hub of the catheter (or under the tubing behind the wings) and cross it over the hub (or wings) to form a chevron with the point distal to the insertion site
- Place a second piece of ½-inch tape across the hub (or wings)
- You may wish to overlap the first chevron with a second chevron for added stability
- Place a sterile dressing over the insertion site
- Secure gauze pad (if used) with 1-inch tape
- Loop the tubing and cover the catheter/needle adapter with a similar piece of 1-inch tape
- Overlap these last two tapes with a labeled piece of 1-inch tape or IV label.

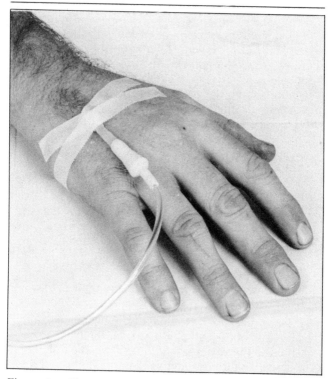

Figure 9-1 Chevron method of taping

3. H method

This method of taping (Figure 9-2) is used with winged needles.

▸ Place a sterile gauze pad over the insertion site
▸ Cover each wing perpendicularly with a piece of 1-inch tape, making sure you also cover an edge of the gauze pad with each piece
▸ Cover the gauze pad and the wings with a piece of 1-inch tape horizontal to the first two, forming a letter H
▸ Loop the tubing and tape the loop in place with 1-inch tape
▸ Overlap these last two tapes with a labeled piece of 1-inch tape or IV label.

4. Alternative H method

With this method, you form the H before applying the sterile gauze pad or other sterile dressing. The crossbar of the H goes over the wings with the dressing on top. This method lets you inspect the insertion site without removing the entire dressing (see Figure 9-3).

5. U method

This method of taping (Figure 9-4) is also used with winged needles or CON devices.

▸ Slip a piece of $\frac{1}{2}$-inch tape, sticky side up, under the catheter hub and fold each end over to make a U (place the ends over the wings of the needle device)
▸ Add a second piece of $\frac{1}{2}$-inch tape over the catheter hub or wings
▸ Place a sterile dressing over the insertion site
▸ If a sterile gauze pad is used, tape the pad in place with a piece of 1-inch tape
▸ Loop the tubing and tape the loop in place with 1-inch tape
▸ Label the dressing.

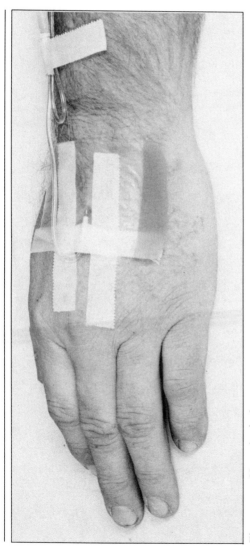

Figure 9-2 H method of taping

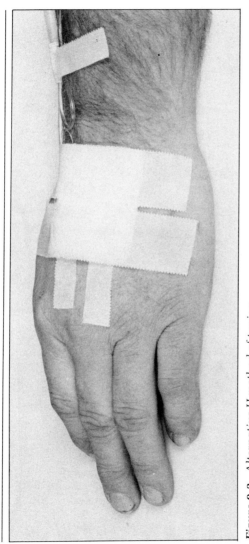

Figure 9-3 Alternative H method of taping

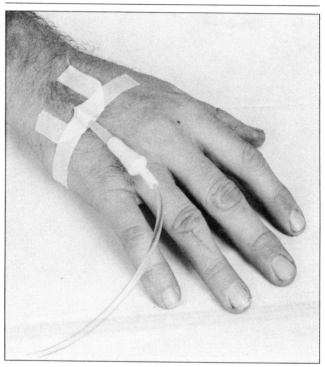

Figure 9-4 U method of taping

6. Scalp-vein method

Scalp venipuncture is done almost exclusively in infants. You'll need to inspect the site more frequently in an infant; this method lets you do so by using a minimum of tape and protection device.

- ▶ Tape down the wings or hub of the venipuncture device with $\frac{1}{4}$-inch or $\frac{1}{2}$-inch tape
- ▶ Place a sterile dressing over the insertion site
- ▶ Make a loop in the tubing and tape the loop in place with $\frac{1}{2}$-inch or 1-inch tape
- ▶ Cover the dressing with labeled $\frac{1}{2}$-inch or 1-inch tape (or, if your institution permits, label the cup in the next step)
- ▶ Cut the bottom off a paper, polystyrene, or medicine cup; cut a slot in the rim; and place the cup over the dressing with the slot over the tubing
- ▶ Tape the cup to the patient's head.

7. Special tips

a. Length. Tapes that go around the patient's extremity may be long enough to meet at the ends. Then, if the patient becomes diaphoretic, the tape won't fall off. But don't continuously wrap the tape around the patient's extremity; it then would act as a tourniquet.

b. Backing. If the IV is placed in an especially hairy area, back the tape with gauze or another piece of tape. Don't shave the area (see Chapter 7).

c. More taping. Don't hesitate to use as much tape as necessary to immobilize the catheter/ needle and stabilize the tubing. For instance, it may be helpful to apply a piece of tape farther up the patient's arm to help absorb tension on the line.

d. Size. If the IV is located in a finger, or if the patient is an infant, you may use smaller tape ($\frac{1}{4}$ inch instead of $\frac{1}{2}$ inch or $\frac{1}{2}$ inch instead of 1 inch).

e. Transparent dressings. Although transparent dressings allow for easy visualization of the site, by eliminating the use of 2×2s, you will still need to stabilize the catheter hub, or wings, before applying the transparent dressing (e.g., Op-Site).

D. BOARDS AND RESTRAINTS

1. When to use a board

Use a board when the infusion is started in the hand, wrist, or antecubital fossa, or when the position of the extremity is important. Use an arm board for the antecubital fossa (and see Chapter 7), a hand board for the hand or wrist, and a tongue depressor for a finger.

2. Positioning the board

Place the patient's hand on the board, palm down with the fingers extending well over the end of the board. Tell the patient to move his/her fingers frequently to help circulation and prevent stiffness.

3. Taping the board

Tape the board both above and below the joint to be immobilized. Don't apply the tape so tightly that it restricts the flow of the IV solution. Back the tape or wrap the patient's arm with gauze where necessary.

4. Restraints

Restraining the patient or wrapping the extremity with gauze may be necessary if the patient is:

▸ Uncooperative
▸ Disoriented

► A child
► Likely to pull the IV out.

Never place a restraint over or above the IV site; it will act as a tourniquet. You may place a restraint below the IV site, or attach the restraint to a board and then tape the patient's hand to the board. Check the patient frequently for irritation and infiltration. In most institutions, soft restraints may be applied without a doctor's order.

E. ADJUSTING THE FLOW RATE

1. Calculation

The orders for administering an IV infusion usually specify the total amount of fluid in liters over the total time in hours, leaving you to figure out how many drops should be infused per minute.

a. Formula. The following formula may be used with any IV tubing or rate of flow:

► Divide the total amount of fluid in milliliters by the total time in minutes to get the amount per minute

► Multiply the amount per minute by the capacity of the drip chamber (10, 15, 20, or 60 drops/ml) to get the number of drops per minute.

To illustrate, let's apply the formula to the following example:

► The orders specify 1 liter (1,000 ml) of fluid to be given in six hours (360 minutes). The drip chamber has a capacity of 15 drops/ml.

$$\frac{1,000}{360} \times 15 = 42 \text{ drops/minute.}$$

b. Shortcut method. A shortcut method may be applied when using a *10, 15, or 20 drops/ml* tubing and the doctor has ordered a specific amount *per hour*. For example:

▶ The orders specify *180 ml per hour* and you are using a *10 drops/ml* tubing. Divide the 180 ml/hour by 6:

$$\frac{180 \text{ ml/hour}}{6} = 30 \text{ drops/minute.}$$

▶ The orders specify *180 ml per hour* and you are using a *15 drops/ml* tubing. Divide the 180 ml/hour by 4:

$$\frac{180 \text{ ml/hour}}{4} = 45 \text{ drops/minute.}$$

▶ The orders specify *180 ml per hour* and you are using a *20 drops/ml* tubing. Divide the 180 ml/hour by 3:

$$\frac{180 \text{ ml/hour}}{3} = 60 \text{ drops/minute.}$$

c. Microdrip tubing. When regulating microdrip tubing (60 drops/ml), there is a direct correlation between the number of milliliters ordered *per hour* and the number of drops per minute the drip rate is set at. For example:

▶ The orders specify *80 ml per hour* and you are using a *60 drops/ml* tubing:

The IV would be set at 80 drops/minute.

d. KVO rates. KVO rates are usually 10 drops/minute (60 ml/hour) with a standard drip set and 20 drops/minute (20 ml/hour) when you use a microdrip set. However, individual policies regarding KVO rates may vary from one institution to another.

2. Regulator clamp

a. Calibrated. Turn the dial to the desired setting.

b. Noncalibrated. Count the number of drops that enter the drip chamber during a one-minute period. Adjust the clamp as needed.

c. Checking. Check the clamp and flow rate periodically, as the clamp may slip or be tampered with.

d. Tampering. Warn the patient not to disturb the clamp and instruct him to tell visitors not to touch it.

F. LABELING AND DOCUMENTATION

Labeling and charting are just as necessary as the other steps in IV therapy. Labeling communicates information to other personnel and serves as a reminder to change tubing and dressings.

1. Labeling the bottle

Write the following information on a label and place it on the bottle upside down, so that it will be right side up when the bottle is hung:

- Patient's name, room number, and ID number
- Dosage—the amount and period of time as ordered by the physician
- Flow rate—the number of drops per minute that you calculated

► Date and time the infusion was started
► Container number—how many bottles the patient has received (if your institution requires this information).

2. Labeling the tubing

Write on a label or piece of tape the date and time the administration set was added. Then fold the label or tape around the tubing to make a tab.

3. Labeling the dressing

Write on a label or piece of 1-inch tape the size and type of venipuncture device, the date and time, and your initials. Place the label or tape on top of the dressing as described in section C above.

4. Charting

The patient's record must include the following information:

► Type and amount of solution hung
► Size and type of venipuncture device
► Date and time
► Site of venipuncture
► Rate of infusion
► Pertinent observations, such as fainting
► Reason for discontinuation of a previous IV (e.g., hematoma, infiltration, phlebitis)
► The name of the person starting the infusion (you).

NOTE: All patient records are legal documents. Always write entries in ink. Never erase, use correction fluid, or cross something out so that it becomes illegible. If you make an error, draw a single line through the incorrect word(s) and write the word "error," the date and time, and your initials above it. Then write in the correct information (see Chapter 20).

CHAPTER **10**

Accessories

A. INFUSION PUMPS AND CONTROLLERS

There are too many makes and models of infusion pumps and controllers to attempt to describe their operation in detail. This section gives only a brief overview of various devices in common use, and their purposes. For detailed instructions on how to operate a device, read the manufacturer's booklet.

1. Advantages

Infusion pumps and controllers can regulate flow rates far more accurately than regulator clamps, and they don't have to be checked and reset as frequently. Controllers and certain types of pumps can deliver fluids much more slowly than manually regulated lines, and they must be used when small amounts of medication are to be administered over relatively long periods. Some pumps are useful for administering viscous fluids, such as blood and lipid emulsions (see Chapters 16 and 18). Finally, many devices contain safety features such as alarms when an air bubble or mechanical malfunction develops.

2. Disadvantages

Some models are fairly difficult to operate and monitor, and all require you to perform additional steps when starting an infusion. Safety features may impart a false sense of security. Not all devices can be converted to gravity operation if they malfunction. Some older, heavier devices unnecessarily limit patients' mobility. Finally, the noise—especially in an intensive-care unit—may have an adverse psychological effect on patients.

3. Types of infusion pumps and volume controllers (see Chapter 5)

a. Syringe pumps. These devices can deliver small volumes of fluids very slowly (as little as 0.01 ml/hour) and are especially useful for purposes such as the following:

▶ Keeping a vein open
▶ Pediatric patients
▶ ICU/CCU settings
▶ Oxytocin infusion to induce labor (special models)
▶ Heparin administration during hemodialysis (special models)
▶ Cardiac catheterization (special models).

b. Peristaltic pumps. There are two kinds of peristaltic pumps: linear and rotary. Certain older models require changing to a different size of tubing in order to adjust the flow rate, a process that increases the chances of contamination. Peristaltic pumps can deliver from 1 to 300 ml/hour, and most models can be converted to gravity flow.

c. Volumetric pumps. Volumetric pumps are the most versatile, with a delivery capacity ranging from 1 to 999 ml/hour. Most types will not pump air—a feature that promotes safety but also requires extra time to remove all air bubbles when the pump is being primed. In general, volumetric pumps are more accurate than syringe and peristaltic pumps. However, because pumps exert a specific force, measured in pounds per square inch, the nurse must check the infusion site frequently for signs of infiltration. Most pumps will not alarm "occlusion" until a substantial amount of fluid has infiltrated the tissues. Another factor to consider in using a pump is the extra cost of the special cartridge and tubing required by most.

d. Infusion-volume controllers. These devices work strictly by gravity. Their value lies in their greater simplicity and safety of operation relative to pumps and their much greater accuracy relative to manually operated clamps. Volume controllers generally deliver between 1 and 300 ml/hour. They cannot be used to deliver viscous fluids. The IV bottle or bag must be hung at least 1 meter above the insertion site, since a volume controller exerts no pumping action. However, since it works by gravity, a volume controller is generally safer to use than a pump: If infiltration occurs, the flow through the volume controller will stop, and alarm, more quickly than when a pump is used.

B. FILTERS

Filters come in different sizes and forms, but they all
have one main purpose: to remove particles from IV
fluids. Particles may be tiny bits of solid material
precipitated from the solution or container, bacteria,
fungi, undissolved drugs, and various other organic
and inorganic impurities. Use a filter whenever:

▶ The patient is to receive a steroid intravenously
▶ An additive is being given
▶ Total parenteral nutrition is being given
▶ Large volumes are being given
▶ The patient is especially susceptible to infection
  (immunosuppressed).

1. Types of filters

a. Depth filters. Depth filters remove
particles of about 5 μm or larger. Because of
their construction, the pore size isn't uniform
and no exact size rating is possible.

b. Membrane filters. As outlined in Chapter
5, membrane filters come in three pore sizes:

▶ 1 to 5 μm—removes particles but does not
  remove bacteria
▶ 0.45 μm—removes most bacteria and
  particulate matter
▶ 0.22 μm—removes all bacteria, fungi,
  yeasts, and particulate matter.

The substance it's made of, as well as the
pore size, determines what a filter can remove.

c. Needle/syringe filters. These are
membrane filters with a pore size of 1 to 5 μm.
They're used to filter medications before
injection into an existing IV line or IV
solution, especially when in-line filters are
not used (see Chapter 11). After you draw up

the medication into the syringe, discard the needle and filter (otherwise, you'll just inject the impurities into the IV line or solution). Attach a new sterile needle, prep the injection port on the tubing or solution with alcohol or povidone-iodine, and then inject the medication into the IV line or solution.

2. Air bubbles

Some membrane filters trap air, while others are air venting. When priming, it's especially important to flush out all air from the line, as any air that does get trapped in the filter will impede the flow of IV solution.

3. In-line vs. add-on filters

Regardless of whether an in-line or add-on filter is used, follow the manufacturer's instructions for priming; some filters need to be inverted while priming, but some do not.

> *a. In-line filters.* In-line, or "final" filters are usually in the 0.22- to 0.45-μm pore-size range. Because they're built into the tubing, a potential source of contamination is eliminated. The disadvantage of an in-line filter is that if an air bubble is trapped or if the filter becomes clogged with particulate matter, the entire tubing must be changed.
>
> *b. Add-on filters.* The greatest disadvantage of an add-on filter is that it introduces two more potential points of contamination. The greatest advantage is flexibility.

4. Flow rate

A very-small-pore-size filter may slow the flow rate. You can partially counteract this effect by hanging the solution higher. Make sure you don't use a filter with a pore size so small that the proper rate of flow can't be maintained. Also, flow rates may begin to slow after the filter has hung for a period of time. This will be particularly noticeable if the patient is receiving multiple doses of medications through the line. The filter is performing its function and trapping all the particulate matter, thus clogging the filter and reducing the rate of flow. The filter and/or tubing must be changed if this should occur.

NOTE: Patients admitted to the emergency room, labor-and-delivery patients, patients going to the operating room, or those experiencing life-threatening situations on the nursing units should *not* have IV lines started with filters. These patients frequently need a "dump" of fluid, which cannot be administered when a filter is in the line.

CHAPTER 11

Additives and admixtures

Patients who are being fed intravenously often
receive their medications intravenously as well. IV
additives can be given in a variety of ways:
simultaneous infusion via a second set, intermittent
infusion via a piggyback set or volume-control
chamber, or admixture with the primary solution. In
addition, medications can be injected directly (see
Chapter 12).

A. SIMULTANEOUS INFUSION

1. Purpose
A second IV set is needed for continuous infusion
of a solution simultaneously with a primary
solution. The second set may be inserted into an
injection port of the primary set, connected by
means of a Y adapter or stopcock, for simultaneous
infusion of two or more solutions. Never give
incompatible substances simultaneously. If you

aren't sure whether two substances are compatible, check. If unable to ascertain their compatibility, do *not* infuse them simultaneously.

2. Equipment

To administer a medication or solution via a second set, you'll need some or all of the following:

- ▸ Filter needle/syringe
- ▸ 18-gauge $1^1/_2$-inch needle
- ▸ Alcohol wipes
- ▸ Bottle/bag of second IV solution
- ▸ Second tubing
- ▸ 20-gauge 1-inch needle
- ▸ $1/_4$- or $1/_2$-inch tape.

3. Procedure for simultaneous infusion

Figure 11-1 shows the setup for simultaneous infusion. The following steps are usually performed by a pharmacist but, in smaller institutions, may still be required of nursing personnel:

- ▸ Remove the cover from the second bottle/bag and swab the stopper with alcohol
- ▸ Draw up the prescribed amount of medication into the filter needle/syringe
- ▸ Discard the needle and filter and replace them with an 18-gauge $1^1/_2$-inch needle
- ▸ Inject the medication into the stopper of the second bottle/bag and gently mix.

If a pharmacist has taken care of the preceding steps, you're responsible for what follows:

- ▸ Spike and hang the bottle/bag and prime the tubing (see Chapter 6)
- ▸ Attach a 20-gauge 1-inch needle to the tubing adapter
- ▸ Swab the injection port of the primary tubing with alcohol and insert the 20-gauge needle (use

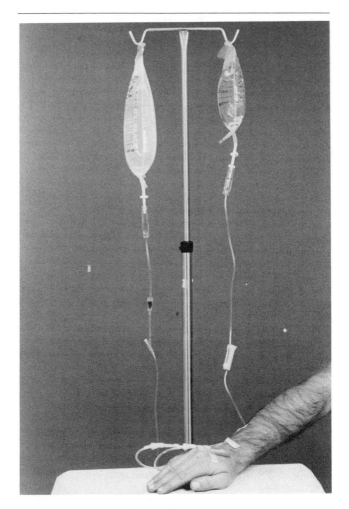

Figure 11-1 Simultaneous infusion

the lower injection port on the primary set, if there is more than one)

▸ Open the clamp on the second line to make sure the solution is flowing freely

▸ Tape the second tubing to the injection port

▸ Regulate the flow rate on the second line

▸ Label the bottle/bag and tubing (see Chapter 13) and chart the procedure.

B. PIGGYBACK

1. Purpose

A piggyback set is used for intermittent infusion of a medication. Intermittent infusion may be necessary to achieve peak blood levels of a medication, or to administer incompatible medications. If the second solution is incompatible with the primary one, flush the tubing with saline before attaching the piggyback to the primary line (see Chapter 13).

2. Equipment

a. Extension hook (usually comes packaged with the piggyback tubing)

b. Bottle/bag of medication/solution

c. Piggyback tubing (shorter than the primary IV tubing)

d. 20-gauge 1-inch needle (usually comes packaged with the piggyback tubing)

e. Alcohol wipes

f. $^1/_4$- or $^1/_2$-inch tape

g. Saline flush. If the two solutions are not compatible, you'll also need the following materials for flushing the primary line before initiating the piggyback infusion:

▸ Bacteriostatic normal (0.9%) saline

▶ Sterile syringe (3 ml)
▶ 20-gauge 1-inch needle.

The procedure for flushing IV lines is outlined in Chapter 13.

3. Procedure for piggyback infusion

Figure 11-2 shows the setup for piggyback infusion. The medication is prepared as for a simultaneous second infusion. Now:

▶ Hang the *primary* bottle/bag on an extension hook
▶ Spike and hang the piggyback bottle/bag and prime the tubing (see Chapter 6)
▶ Attach a 20-gauge 1-inch needle to the tubing adapter, if one not already built into it by the manufacturer
▶ Swab the piggyback (upper, backchecked) port of the primary tubing with alcohol
▶ If the two solutions are incompatible, flush the tubing below the injection port with saline (see Chapter 13)
▶ Insert the 20-gauge needle in the piggyback port and fully open the clamp on the piggyback set
▶ Tape the piggyback tubing to the injection port
▶ Regulate the flow rate with the regulator clamp on the tubing of the primary solution
▶ Label the bottle/bag and tubing (see Chapter 13) and chart the procedure.

C. VOLUME-CONTROL CHAMBERS

1. Purpose

A volume-control chamber, also called a fluid chamber, burette, Volutrol, Soluset, or Buretrol, is used instead of a piggyback set for intermittent infusion when precise control of flow rate is necessary, as when a small amount of medication

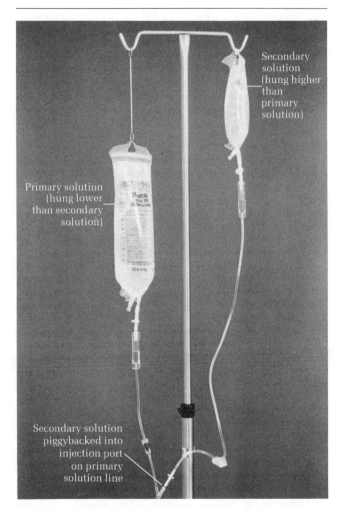

Figure 11-2 Piggyback infusion

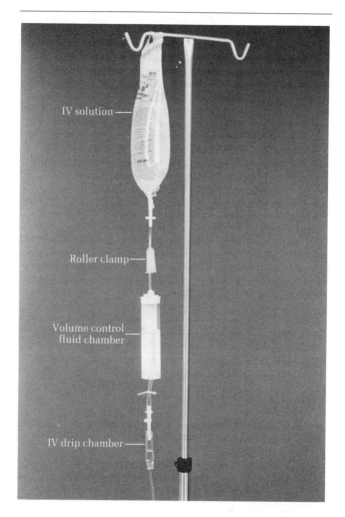

Figure 11-3 Volume-controlled infusion

is to be infused over a long period. A volume-control set is often used as the primary line for infants and small children.

2. Equipment

a. Additional equipment. The additional equipment is the same as for a simultaneous infusion (section A) except that the second tubing contains a volume-control chamber.

b. Drip rate. Most volume-control chambers are made to deliver 60 (microdrip) drops/ml.

c. Filters. Some volume-control chambers contain either a floating-valve filter or a membrane filter. The procedures for priming the drip chambers for the two types of filters are different. Consult the manufacturer's directions for priming these devices.

3. Procedure for volume-controlled infusion

Figure 11-3 shows the setup for volume-controlled infusion.

a. Beginning steps. Draw up the medication, spike and hang the bottle/bag, with all clamps closed, as for a simultaneous infusion, and then prime.

b. Priming with a floating-valve filter

► Open the upper clamp and squeeze the volume-control chamber until it's about half full; then close the upper clamp

► Squeeze the drip chamber until it's about half full.

c. Priming with a membrane filter

► Open the upper clamps and fill the volume-control chamber halfway (don't squeeze it); then close both upper clamps

► Open the lower clamp, squeeze the drip chamber flat, and close the clamp. Then release the drip chamber and allow it to fill about halfway. This procedure is easily remembered by associating it with OSCAR:

*O*pen

*S*queeze

*C*lose

*A*nd

*R*elease

► Repeat the last step, if necessary, until the drip chamber is at least half full.

d. Remaining procedure

► Attach a 20-gauge needle to the needle adapter

► Open the lower clamp, prime the tubing, and close the clamp

► Swab the injection port of the fluid chamber with alcohol

► Inject medication into the volume-control chamber

► Open the upper clamp, let the prescribed quantity of solution run into the volume-control chamber, and close the upper clamp

► Gently mix the medication and solution

► Swab the injection port on the primary line with an alcohol wipe

► Attach the second tubing to the lower port on the primary line

► Clamp off the primary line or set it at KVO

► Set the lower clamp on the volume-control set at the prescribed flow rate

► Tape the second tubing to the injection port

► Label the second bottle/bag and volume-control chamber (see Chapter 13) and chart the procedure.

NOTE: A volume-control infusion line may also be used as the primary IV line.

D. ADMIXTURE WITH PRIMARY SOLUTION

1. Purpose
By mixing one or more drugs with the primary solution, you avoid several possibilities of contamination and considerably simplify administration and maintenance of the infusion. Admixture is possible only with compatible substances that are to be infused at the same rate.

2. Equipment
For each medication you add to the IV solution, if your institution's pharmacy doesn't perform this function, you'll need the following:

▶ Filter needle/syringe
▶ Small-gauge (large-bore) 1½-inch needle
▶ Prescribed amount of drug in correct diluent.

Other devices, such as double-headed pins and ampoule-transfer siphons, are available for specialized applications.

3. Procedure
a. Injecting medication before spiking.
Again, the first four steps are increasingly performed by hospital pharmacies, which are better equipped than nursing stations.

▶ Draw the medication into the syringe
▶ Discard the needle and filter and replace with a small-gauge 1½-inch needle
▶ Remove the cap from the bottle/bag and swab the stopper with alcohol
▶ Inject the medication into the bottle/bag through the stopper and mix gently
▶ Before you administer the medication, inspect the solution for cloudiness,

particles, color change, foaming, and other signs that something is wrong

▸ Label the bottle/bag (see Chapter 13) and chart the procedure.

b. Injecting medication into a hanging bottle/bag. Always make sure there's enough solution in the hanging container to dilute the drug sufficiently. If there isn't, hang a fresh container. Always swab the injection port with alcohol before injecting medication. And always clamp off the tubing before you inject any drug; otherwise the patient may receive a bolus of the drug.

▸ Nonvented bottle—remove the vent on the tubing, inject the medication into the vent port, and replace the vent (don't touch either end of the vent)

▸ Vented bottle—inject the medication into the triangle on the stopper

▸ Bag—inject the medication into the port provided for that purpose

▸ Mix the medication and solution gently by agitating the bottle/bag; don't pull on the tubing

▸ Label the bottle/bag (see Chapter 13) and chart the procedure.

Direct IV injection

Certain drugs work best when injected directly into the vein rather than infused, whether or not the patient has an IV infusion running at the time. Medications may be injected rapidly or slowly, over a period of several minutes, through a variety of routes. The route depends partly on whether the medication is compatible with the primary solution. State and institutional regulations may prohibit IV injections by nurses who aren't members of special teams or units (see Chapter 20), or may permit nurses to inject only certain drugs intravenously.

A. INJECTION DIRECTLY INTO A VEIN

IV medications may be injected directly into a vein, by IV bolus or push, when it is important for the patient to receive a large dose of medication fast, when the patient doesn't have an infusion running, or when it is impractical to inject medication through an existing line.

▶ *IV bolus:* The manual administration directly into a vein or IV tubing at a rate of 1 ml/30 seconds or less

▶ *IV push:* The manual administration directly into a vein or IV tubing at a rate of 1 ml/minute or greater.

1. Equipment

a. Rapid injection (IV bolus). For injection all at once or very rapidly, you will need:

▶ Tourniquet
▶ Filter needle/syringe or prefilled syringe supplied by a drug manufacturer
▶ Straight needle or winged needle
▶ Povidone-iodine or alcohol wipe
▶ Sterile gauze pads.

b. Prolonged injection (IV push). An alternative to inserting a needle directly attached to the syringe is the use of a winged-needle unit with the catheter attached to the syringe. The winged needle, being smaller and steadier than the syringe needle, is less likely to damage or perforate the vein over a period of several minutes. Also, because the tension is on the catheter rather than on your hand, a winged-needle unit is more comfortable for both you and the patient. For this procedure you'll need:

▶ Tourniquet
▶ Filter needle/syringe or prefilled syringe supplied by a drug manufacturer
▶ Winged-needle set
▶ Povidone-iodine or alcohol wipe
▶ Sterile gauze pads
▶ Tape.

2. Procedure

a. Rapid injection (IV bolus)

▸ Draw up the medication into the filter needle/syringe if not already supplied in a filled syringe

▸ Discard the needle and filter and replace with the straight needle or winged needle

▸ Choose a vein, cleanse the insertion site with povidone-iodine or alcohol, and wipe with a gauze pad

▸ Perform venipuncture as described in Chapter 8

▸ If you're using a winged needle, place a piece of tape over the wings to stabilize the device

▸ Inject the medication with slow, even pressure—do not force the plunger

▸ Observe the patient closely for signs of adverse reaction

▸ Remove the tape, if any

▸ Place a sterile gauze pad over the site as you withdraw the needle

▸ Press the pad gently on the insertion site for one minute or until bleeding stops

▸ Cover the site with a sterile gauze pad or Band-Aid

▸ Chart the procedure.

b. Prolonged injection (IV push)

▸ Draw up the medication into the filter needle/syringe if not already supplied in a filled syringe

▸ Disconnect and discard the needle and filter and attach the syringe to the catheter of the winged-needle set

▸ Choose a vein and prep the insertion site as described above

- Perform venipuncture as described in Chapter 8
- Flatten the wings of the needle and place a piece of tape over the wings to stabilize the device
- Inject the medication over the designated time period and observe the patient closely for signs of a reaction
- Remove the tape
- Place a sterile gauze pad over the insertion site as you withdraw the needle
- Press the pad gently on the insertion site for one minute or until bleeding stops
- Cover the site with a sterile gauze pad or Band-Aid
- Chart the procedure.

B. INJECTION THROUGH LOWER PORT OF TUBING

1. Purpose

This is the most common route, and the easiest to use, in patients who already have an IV infusion. Incompatible medications can be given directly into the IV line as long as the tubing is flushed with saline before and after injection of the incompatible substance (see Chapter 13).

2. Equipment

- Filter needle/syringe
- Prescribed medication
- Large-gauge (small-bore) needle
- Alcohol wipes.

3. Procedure

Figure 12-1 shows the procedure for IV push into the injection port on IV tubing.

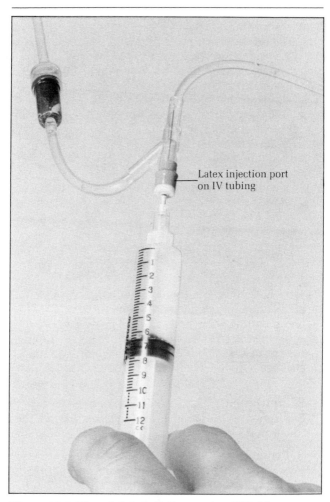

Latex injection port
on IV tubing

Figure 12-1 IV push into injection port on IV tubing

- Draw up the appropriate amount of medication with a filter needle/syringe
- Discard the needle and filter and replace with a large-gauge needle
- Swab the lower injection port with alcohol and insert the needle
- Clamp off the tubing above the port
- If necessary, flush the tubing below the port with saline (see Chapter 13)
- Aspirate for blood
- Inject the medication
- If necessary, flush again
- Open the clamp and regulate the flow rate
- Chart the procedure.

C. INJECTION THROUGH A FLASHBULB OR STOPCOCK

1. Purpose
This method is equally useful whether the medication to be injected is compatible or incompatible with large-volume parenteral solutions, as it doesn't involve flushing the tubing. A stopcock is used if there's no flashbulb. In the absence of both a flashbulb and stopcock, the medication may be injected directly into the vein.

2. Equipment
Equipment is the same as for injection through the lower port of the tubing.

3. Procedure
Procedure is also the same as for injection through the lower port of the tubing, except that the flashbulb or port on the stopcock is used and the tubing is not flushed (see Figures 12-2 and 12-3).

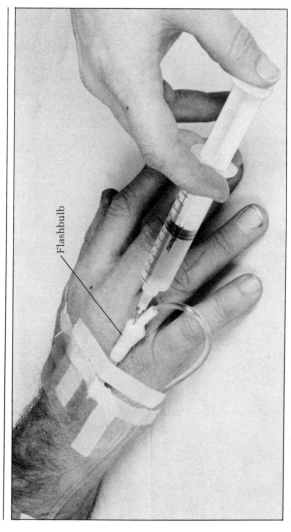

Flashbulb

Figure 12-2 IV push through flashbulb in IV tubing

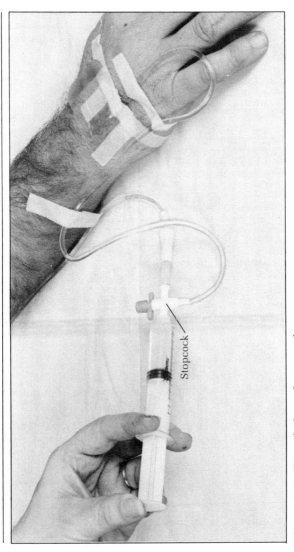

Stopcock

Figure 12-3 IV push through stopcock

D. INJECTION THROUGH A HEPARIN LOCK OR INTERMITTENT-INFUSION RESERVOIR

1. Purpose

A heparin lock or intermittent-infusion reservoir is used when a patient needs intermittent infusion or slow injection of medication but doesn't require a constant infusion. It keeps the vein open by preventing clotting but has the added advantages of allowing the patient greater mobility than a continuous hookup and of reducing the risk of fluid overload. A heparin lock or intermittent-infusion reservoir can also be used for drawing blood samples.

NOTE: Explain to the patient why he/she will have the device inserted, and make sure the patient understands that it must be kept clean and dry and protected from trauma.

2. Equipment

A standard winged-needle set or CON can be converted to a heparin lock by inserting a special adapter plug. If you have a choice, a CON is preferable to a winged-needle device.

- ▸ Tourniquet
- ▸ Winged-needle or CON device
- ▸ Intermittent-infusion adapter plug (PRN adapter)—winged-needle and CON devices are also available with pre-attached intermittent-infusion adapter plugs
- ▸ Sterile dressing (gauze pad, Band-Aid, or transparent dressing)
- ▸ Alcohol and povidone-iodine wipes
- ▸ Tuberculin syringe, or prefilled cartridge, containing 0.5 to 1.0 ml of heparin saline flush solution (1:10 to 1:100 or 1:1,000 units of heparin

saline flush solution may be used as stipulated by your hospital's policy)
▸ 3-ml syringe containing normal (0.9%) saline, attached to a 22- or 25-gauge needle
▸ Antimicrobial ointment (if it's required by your institution)
▸ $\frac{1}{2}$- and 1-inch tape.

3. Starting a heparin lock
▸ Choose a vein and prep the patient as described in Chapter 7
▸ Wipe the rubber injection port of the reservoir with alcohol
▸ Flush the reservoir with 1 ml of normal saline and leave the needle, with syringe attached, in the reservoir
▸ With the winged-needle or CON device, perform venipuncture as described in Chapter 8 and check for blood return
▸ Withdraw the stylet from the CON device, or the venting plug from the winged-needle device, and attach the PRN adapter to the hub of the CON or winged-needle device
▸ Tape the device securely
▸ Inject 2 ml of normal saline through the reservoir and observe the site for infiltration; if there's none, withdraw the needle/syringe
▸ Wipe the port with alcohol, inject medication if an injectable dose is scheduled, and flush out any remaining medication with saline
▸ Apply antimicrobial ointment, such as povidone-iodine, to the venipuncture site, if required by your hospital's policy, and apply a sterile dressing as described in Chapter 9
▸ Swab the injection port with alcohol
▸ Inject the heparin saline flush solution
▸ Label the site and chart the procedure.

4. Administering medications by means of a heparin lock

a. Injection. Figure 12-4 shows the procedure for IV push through a heparin lock.

- ▸ Swab the injection port with alcohol
- ▸ Draw up the medication in a syringe
- ▸ Draw up 0.5 to 1.0 ml of heparin saline flush solution in a tuberculin syringe (1:10 to 1:100 or 1:1,000 units of heparin saline flush solution may be used according to your hospital's policy)
- ▸ Draw up 3 ml of normal saline in a syringe with a 22- or 25-gauge needle
- ▸ Insert the needle with the normal saline into the injection port and aspirate for blood
- ▸ Flush the reservoir with saline and remove the needle and syringe
- ▸ Swab the injection port with alcohol
- ▸ Insert the needle with the medication into the injection port and inject the medication at the prescribed rate
- ▸ Remove the medication needle and syringe
- ▸ Swab the injection port with alcohol
- ▸ Repeat the injection of saline flush for each drug to be administered
- ▸ Inject from 0.5 to 1 ml of heparin saline flush solution
- ▸ Observe the patient for a possible reaction and chart the procedure.

b. Infusion. Figure 12-5 shows an IV infusion attached to a heparin lock.

- ▸ Set up the necessary equipment and prime it as described in Chapter 6
- ▸ Swab the injection port with alcohol

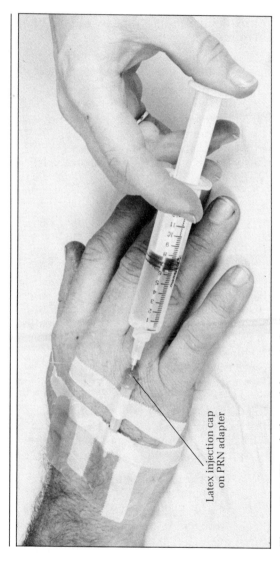

Latex injection cap
on PRN adapter

Figure 12-4 IV push through heparin lock

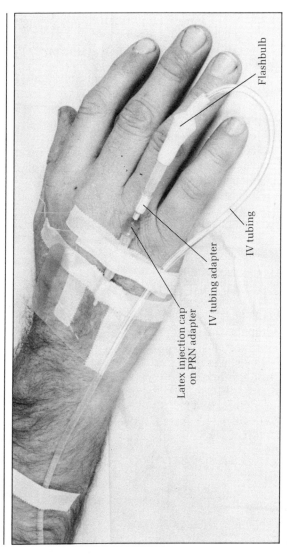

Figure 12-5 IV infusion attached to heparin lock

- ► Draw up 3 ml of normal saline in a syringe with a 22- or 25-gauge needle
- ► Insert the needle into the injection port and aspirate for blood
- ► Flush the reservoir with saline and remove the needle and syringe
- ► Swab the injection port with alcohol
- ► Attach a sterile needle to the IV tubing and insert the needle into the injection port
- ► Regulate the flow rate
- ► Label the bottle/bag appropriately and chart the procedure
- ► After the infusion has ended, detach the IV administration set, flush the reservoir with 3 ml of saline, and inject 0.5 to 1 ml of heparin saline flush solution.

E. ADVANTAGES OF
DIRECT IV INJECTION

The advantages of direct IV injection are:

- ► Immediate peak blood levels may be achieved
- ► It is fast and easy to administer, particularly in an emergency situation
- ► Less fluid volume is required than for IV piggyback or primary solution
- ► It may be given if PO or IM route is contraindicated
- ► It may be the desired route if the drug would be incompatible with other IV drugs or solutions being infused.

F. DISADVANTAGES OF DIRECT IV INJECTION

The disadvantages of direct IV injection include the following:

- Immediate peak blood levels may be achieved—the entire dose is on board and, consequently, reactions will tend to be more severe
- It may cause venous irritation—many of the drugs are fairly concentrated and irritate the vein intima
- It may be time consuming—IV push drugs may take several minutes to administer
- If a patient's circulatory system is compromised (i.e., in an arrest), the risk of intra-arterial injection is greatly increased ("normal" landmarks and distinguishing signs are absent); observation must be intensified to prevent serious consequences
- The medication can't be given by direct IV injection if it needs to be diluted in a large amount of solute. It would then be best to give the drug by primary or piggyback infusion.

G. POSSIBLE COMPLICATIONS OF DIRECT IV INJECTION

1. Drugs that frequently cause severe reaction

a. CNS depressants. These include tranquilizers, analgesics, narcotics.

b. Anti-inflammatory agents

c. Anesthetics

d. Antibiotics

e. Antineoplastics

f. Anticonvulsants

2. Possible side effects

a. Cardiac arrhythmias

b. GI upset. With some drugs, this may be an early warning of reaching toxic levels.

c. CNS depression. Side effects include drowsiness, mental confusion, hypotension, respiratory depression.

d. GU symptoms

e. Neurological symptoms

f. Extravasation. Some of the drugs that are particularly irritating to soft tissues on infiltration include:

- Dopamine
- Dilantin
- Mannitol
- Valium
- Phenobarbital
- Digoxin
- Dextrose (greater than 10%)
- Anti-inflammatory agents
- Antineoplastics
- Vasoconstrictors.

H. ANTIDOTES

Antidotes for various drug reactions due to direct injection include:

- Diphenhydramine (Benadryl)—for allergic rash or phenothiazine reaction
- Epinephrine—for allergic anaphylactoid respiratory reactions
- Phentolamine (Regitine)—for adverse reaction to vasoconstrictors
- Naloxone (Narcan)—for reaction to narcotics

▶ Protamine sulfate—for reaction to heparin
▶ Antineoplastics reaction—sodium thiosulfate for mechlorethamine (Mustargen); sodium bicarbonate for doxorubicin (Adriamycin); hyaluronidase (Wydase) for vincristine (Oncovin) and vinblastine (Velban).

I. BASIC CONSIDERATIONS

The basic considerations for administering any drug directly into a patient's venous system must include:

1. Application of the five R's
▶ Right patient
▶ Right drug
▶ Right dose
▶ Right route
▶ Right time.

2. Knowledge of the patient's condition and medical history
▶ Be aware of the patient's condition *before* administering the medication
▶ Know the patient's history, allergies, and/or possible contraindications for using the drug, e.g., propranolol (Inderal) is indicated for the treatment of tachycardia but is contraindicated for use with asthmatic patients.

3. Following correct procedure
Follow correct procedure (as stated earlier in this chapter), utilizing aseptic technique.

CHAPTER 13

Compatibility of IV solutions

This chapter can't begin to list all drug and IV solution incompatibilities; that would take a book in itself. Rather, here are some general guidelines to follow. For information about specific drugs and IV solutions, you may consult reference sources such as those listed in section D.

A. LABELING

Whenever you add medication to an IV solution, you must label the bottle/bag with the following pertinent information:

- ► Name of patient
- ► Patient's ID or hospital number
- ► Patient's room number and bed
- ► Name of medication
- ► Amount and strength of medication
- ► Expiration date of medication
- ► Diluent or reconstitution medium, if any

- ▶ Date and time medication was added
- ▶ Name of IV solution
- ▶ Flow rate
- ▶ Your name or initials as required by institutional policy.

B. TYPES OF INCOMPATIBILITIES

There are a limited number of references on intravenous incompatibilities (see section D), and much remains unknown. For those reasons, it is critical for the nurse to understand some of the basic or underlying mechanisms of incompatibilities and to be able to identify potential problems that can be researched for more definitive answers or referred to the IV admixture pharmacy service, if one exists, in the hospital. Intravenous incompatibilities may result from undesirable chemical or physical phenomena when two or more intravenous medications come into contact with each other. In general, incompatibilities can be divided into two categories, therapeutic and pharmaceutical. Pharmaceutical incompatibilities can be further divided into physical and chemical categories.

1. Therapeutic incompatibilities
Therapeutic incompatibilities result when two or more incompatible drugs are combined, which produces a response completely different in nature or in intensity from that expected. An example of such a reaction is in the mixture of an aminoglycoside (gentamicin) and a penicillin (carbenicillin, ticarcillin) in the same bottle or in the infusion of the two drugs simultaneously in the same primary tubing. A chemical reaction between the two drugs results, causing inactivation

of the aminoglycoside and thus preventing the patient from receiving the full benefit of the antibiotic. A more general example deals with the combination of a bacteriostatic and a bactericidal antibiotic. Whether these antibiotics are infused together or separately, a therapeutic incompatibility results, not from the chemical characteristics of each drug, but from their pharmacologic effects. A bacteriostatic antibiotic (e.g., chloramphenicol) inhibits bacterial growth, whereas a bactericidal antibiotic (e.g., penicillin) kills bacteria. Since bactericidal antibiotics are only effective against multiplying bacteria, bacteriostatic antibiotics may inhibit the antibacterial effect of the bactericidal antibiotic.

2. Pharmaceutical incompatibilities

a. Physical incompatibilities. Physical incompatibilities may result from the inability of a drug to dissolve in a solution or from the combination of two drugs, which forms a complex or precipitate that is insoluble and is visualized as a precipitate or haze. On occasion such a reaction may result in a color change of the solution or the evolution of gas in the admixture. Examples of physical incompatibilities are Valium mixed in D_5W and phenytoin sodium added to an aqueous solution with an acidic pH.

b. Chemical incompatibilities. Chemical incompatibilities result from reactions that are often manifested in both a physical and a therapeutic incompatibility. A chemical incompatibility may result in a therapeutic incompatibility without the formation of visual physical evidence. An example is the hydrolysis of drugs. Penicillin in water is eventually inactivated without visual evidence. The chemical reaction between acidic and basic drugs is the most common source of chemical incompatibility. Such a combination may result in a new pH of the solution and a consequent instability of one of the drugs. Examples include ampicillin in D_5W stored at room temperature for more than four hours prior to administration and the oxidation of epinephrine in alkaline solutions when exposed to light.

C. GENERAL GUIDELINES

1. Diluent
Does the medication have its own diluent, as do drugs such as diazepam (Valium)? If it does, it's probably incompatible with other medications or IV solutions.

2. Printed precautions
Does the package insert or label contain precautions on mixing the medication, as with drugs such as erythromycin lactobionate (Erythrocin Lactobionate-IV) or nitroprusside (Nipride)? If so, read the directions carefully.

3. Colloids
Colloids like amphotericin B (Fungizone) are likely to "salt out" (precipitate) in the presence of electrolytes such as sodium chloride (saline) and bacteriostatic agents such as benzyl alcohol.

4. Blood
Never mix blood or blood products with anything. The protein in blood may bind to other agents and destroy their effectiveness. Even more important, you risk coagulation or lysis of the cells.

5. Antibiotics

a. Drug interactions. Try to avoid mixing antibiotics in the same solution, as they're likely to interact. For example, tetracyclines interfere with the bactericidal action of penicillins; carbenicillin or ticarcillin inactivates gentamicin or tobramycin.

b. Hydrolysis. Does the medication look, smell, or sound like one of the penicillins—for example, ampicillin (Alpen-N, Amcill-S, Penbritin-S, Polycillin-N), carbenicillin (Geopen, Pyopen), or methicillin (Dimocillin, Staphcillin)? These antibiotics are easily hydrolyzed by either acids or bases.

6. Calcium

Calcium is an electrolyte and is present in many commonly used parenteral solutions (e.g., lactated Ringer's solution). At an alkaline pH it will be precipitated out of solution, especially when drugs such as cephalothin sodium (Keflin), sodium bicarbonate, and potassium phosphate are added to the solution.

7. Mixing intravenous admixtures (acidity and alkalinity)

Add one drug at a time to the large-volume parenteral solution, mix it thoroughly, and then examine it visually. Some visual incompatibilities are concentration dependent and may require a certain amount of time or concentration before appearing. It is a good idea to add the most concentrated or most soluble additive to the solution first. The more dilute the drug is, the less likely that acid-base interactions will occur. Any medication with a very high pH (alkaline) or low pH (acid) is likely to cause compatibility problems.

8. Precipitates

Some precipitates are very fine and dispersed, making them very difficult to detect. This is especially true if the solution is colored, as when multivitamins or riboflavin are added. In such cases, add the color-producing drug last in order to be able to visualize the solution. For example, Valium added to a large-volume parenteral is very critical since Valium's solubility in water is low. If Valium's solubility is exceeded, a fine yellow precipitate results. The intense yellow color of multivitamins may mask the Valium precipitate if Valium is added to the solution first.

9. Phenol red

An orange solution that is not a vitamin may contain phenol red, which is sensitive to alkaline pH. It may not be disconcerting to you to mix an additive containing phenol red (e.g., potassium chloride, magnesium chloride, or calcium chloride) with a compatible basic drug (e.g., ampicillin), but the resulting magenta color may create panic among patients, physicians, and other nurses.

10. Rules of thumb

a. Pharmacologic groups of drugs (families) usually react in a similar manner. If you know of an incompatibility with one drug, most likely the same is true for the other drugs in that group.

b. If you aren't sure about the compatibility of drugs to be mixed, do not proceed before either contacting someone who can provide you with an answer or researching an answer yourself. If you are unable to find out about the compatibility, do *not* mix them.

D. SOURCES OF INFORMATION ON DRUG COMPATIBILITY

Your hospital pharmacist should be a good source of information. Alternatively, you may consult published materials such as the following:

▶ American Hospital Formulary Service
▶ *Drug Interactions Index* by Fred Lerman and Robert T. Weibert (Medical Economics, 1982)
▶ *A Guide to I.V. Admixture Compatibility* (3rd edition; Medical Economics, 1980)
▶ *Intravenous Medications* by Diane Proctor Sager and Suzanne Kovarovic Bomar (Lippincott, 1980)
▶ *Physicians' Desk Reference* (Medical Economics; published yearly)
▶ *Pocket Guide to Injectable Drugs* by L. A. Trissel (American Society of Hospital Pharmacists, 1981).

E. FLUSHING IV LINES

1. Purpose
Flushing helps prevent incompatible substances from coming into contact with each other. Flush with sterile nonpyrogenic normal saline (0.9%) after each incompatible medication you inject through the IV tubing or the intermittent-infusion reservoir.

2. Equipment
▶ Sterile syringe containing 2 to 3 ml of sterile nonpyrogenic normal saline (0.9%)
▶ Small needle
▶ Alcohol wipes.

3. Procedure
▶ Swab the injection port with alcohol
▶ Clamp or pinch off the IV tubing above the injection port

► Inject the saline slowly through the injection port (don't force it)
► If necessary, aspirate and try again
► Withdraw the needle and check for free flow of IV fluid.

CHAPTER **14**

Changing and discontinuing IV infusions

When handling IV equipment, maintain sterile technique at all times. If you have any doubt about the sterility of any piece of equipment, discard it.

A. CHANGING IV SOLUTION CONTAINERS

1. Frequency
Change containers at least every 24 hours, and more often according to a physician's orders. It isn't necessary to wait for the bottle/bag to be emptied of the last drop of solution before you change it.

2. Procedure
For spiking and priming technique, see Chapter 6.

▶ Make sure the drip chamber under the old container is at least half full
▶ Close the regulator clamp to a KVO rate

▶ Remove the protective cap from the new container. If using a bottle, wipe the rubber stopper on the bottle with an alcohol wipe
▶ Remove the old container from the IV pole
▶ Remove the spike from the old container and insert it in the new one
▶ Hang the new container and label it
▶ Regulate the flow rate
▶ Drain any remaining solution from the old container and discard it in the proper receptacle
▶ Chart the procedure.

B. CHANGING IV ADMINISTRATION SETS AND DRESSINGS

1. Frequency
Change tubing and dressings at least every 24 to 48 hours. If possible, time the change to coincide with changes of containers and needle or catheter. However, if a patient is admitted with an IV already running, you may need to connect new tubing and a new container to the catheter/needle already in place. Always change the administration set after administering blood. If transparent dressings are used, they need not be changed until the IV site is changed, unless they become wet or contaminated.

2. Procedure
▶ Close the regulator clamp on the new tubing
▶ Remove the protective cover or cap from the new container. If a bottle is used, wipe the stopper with an alcohol wipe
▶ Spike the container
▶ Hang the new container and prime the tubing (see Chapter 6)
▶ If the dressing is to be changed, hold the catheter/needle in place with one hand and

remove the old dressing from the IV site, being careful not to dislodge or wiggle the catheter/needle unnecessarily
- ▶ Cleanse the insertion site with povidone-iodine and let it dry. You may also apply antimicrobial ointment, if required by your hospital's policy
- ▶ Place a large sterile gauze pad or alcohol wipe under the hub and adapter
- ▶ Close the regulator clamp on the old IV tubing
- ▶ With one hand holding the catheter/needle, grasp the hub and carefully remove the old tubing adapter
- ▶ Remove the protective cap from the new tubing and attach the new adapter to the hub
- ▶ Remove the gauze pad or alcohol wipe and clean the area of any blood or fluid that may have spilled during the procedure
- ▶ Apply a new dressing
- ▶ Loop the tubing and tape it to the patient's skin
- ▶ Regulate the flow rate
- ▶ Label the new container, tubing, and dressing
- ▶ Drain any remaining solution from the old container and tubing and discard them in the designated receptacle along with the old dressing
- ▶ Chart the procedure.

C. CHANGING IV CATHETERS/NEEDLES

Unless the patient is running short of acceptable new sites, an IV infusion should be moved every 48 to 72 hours. This, of course, involves a completely new prep, venipuncture, and infusion start, which are covered in Chapters 7, 8, and 9, respectively. If the site needs to be extended beyond 72 hours because of limited venous access, the physician should be notified and an order for the infusion to continue at that site should be obtained and documented in the patient's record. The infusion site should then be watched even more closely and the IV removed at the first sign of irritation, infiltration, and/or phlebitis.

D. CHANGING STOPCOCKS

Stopcocks should be changed every 24 to 48 hours, at the same time tubing is changed. If you change the tubing because you suspect it's contaminated, you must also change the stopcock. Once the injection-port cover is removed, consider the port contaminated; don't use it again.

E. USING AN OBTURATOR

1. Purpose
When an infusion must be discontinued and the tubing disconnected for a short period, as when a patient is taken for X-rays or a brief procedure, you may keep the catheter open with an obturator. NOTE: An obturator is used only for short periods; don't use one between intermittent infusions. Never use the same obturator more than once; after one use, it's contaminated.

2. Procedure
▶ Disconnect the tubing (see section B)
▶ Insert the obturator into the catheter
▶ Twist the cap until it clicks shut
▶ Tape the obturator to the patient's skin.

F. DISCONTINUING AN INFUSION

1. Routine removal
▶ Remove the outer tape and the dressing
▶ Stabilize the catheter/needle with one hand and carefully remove the tape (avoid moving the catheter/needle inside the vein)

▶ Press gently on the puncture site with a sterile gauze pad

▶ Slowly withdraw the catheter/needle in line with the vein (see Figure 14-1)

▶ Press firmly on the site for at least 30 seconds, or until bleeding stops, to avoid a hematoma. You may elevate the limb during the time digital pressure is being applied

▶ Cover the site with a sterile gauze pad or a sterile Band-Aid

▶ Chart the procedure

▶ Empty any remaining solution from the container and tubing and discard them, along with the dressing and catheter/needle, in the designated receptacles.

2. Removal when there's a problem with the infusion

a. Failure to flow well. Try to reestablish good flow by techniques like these:

▶ Repositioning the catheter

▶ Squeezing the tubing

▶ Hanging the bottle/bag higher

▶ Flushing with saline and aspirating.

If a filter is used, it may be clogged and thus need to be changed. If necessary, get help from someone more experienced—such as your institution's IV team.

b. Infiltration or clotting. If you're unable to reestablish good flow by any of the methods recommended above, suspect infiltration or a clot in the catheter—even if no signs of these problems are evident. If you suspect the site may have been infiltrated with a drug that could be damaging to the soft tissues, close the regulator clamp on the IV tubing but do *not*

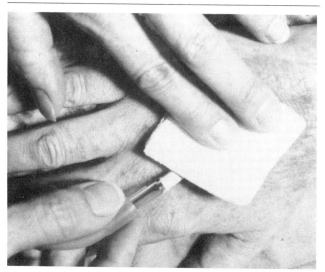

Figure 14-1 *Discontinuing an infusion*

remove the catheter/needle. Contact the IV therapy specialist on duty or the pharmacist for possible action. If the infiltration involves a plain solution or medication that won't damage soft tissues, discontinue the infusion at once and start again in another vein.

c. Redness, soreness, or phlebitis. If an IV site is red, sore, or phlebotic, the line must be discontinued. If a bacterial infection is suspected, culture the site (see Chapter 19) before discontinuing the infusion. If necessary, call on someone more experienced for help. And, to help the healing process and make the patient more comfortable, apply warm, moist compresses to the area.

d. Charting and follow-up. Chart any problems you find when discontinuing an infusion, and alert the appropriate personnel as to the need for continued observation of the puncture site.

G. DISPOSAL OF USED EQUIPMENT

All used IV equipment, from the bottle/bag on down, is contaminated. Therefore, you can't just drop it in the nearest wastebasket. For the protection of curious visitors and of all personnel who participate in waste disposal, used IV equipment must be discarded in special receptacles.

1. Bottles, bags, and tubing
These should be drained and placed in the designated receptacle.

2. Needles
Remove the old needle from the adapter by cutting or breaking it off. Place the old needle in a receptacle specifically designated for contaminated needles. If you accidentally pierce your skin with a contaminated needle, report the incident.

3. Syringes
If possible, crush a used syringe; if not, remove the rubber tip of the plunger. Discard the syringe in the specifically designated receptacle.

CHAPTER **15**

Monitoring IV infusions

Many things can go wrong with an IV infusion. Some complications of IV therapy can quickly become fatal. That's why it's important to check infusions frequently—at least hourly, and more often if a hypertonic solution or a drug is being infused or if the patient is very young, old, or debilitated.

A. PROBLEMS WITH FLOW RATE

1. Runaway IV

a. What may happen. A clamp may slip, or the patient or a visitor may open a clamp. The resulting too-rapid infusion might not do harm, but it could have drastic, even fatal, consequences:

- ▸ Circulatory overload, leading to congestive heart failure and pulmonary edema
- ▸ Toxic overdose of a medication infused faster than the body can metabolize it.

b. Intervention. If you observe signs of congestive heart failure or pulmonary edema—rapid, labored breathing, rapid pulse, increased blood pressure, distended neck veins—slow the infusion to its minimum rate, place the patient in high Fowler's position, and call a physician. If you observe signs of shock or anaphylaxis, replace the infusion with normal (0.9%) saline and call a physician. The saline infusion keeps the vein open and helps counteract the effects of shock on the circulatory volume.

c. Suggestions for prevention

▶ Know your patient's cardiovascular status and medical history

▶ Monitor your patient's intake and output carefully

▶ Notify the physician if your patient appears unable to handle the fluid volume

▶ Check the IV infusion frequently for correct flow rate.

2. Obstructed or irregular flow

a. What may happen. A solution may refuse to flow at the prescribed rate, or may stop entirely, for any of several reasons:

▶ The tourniquet may have been left on the patient's arm

▶ The catheter/needle may be pushed against the vein wall

▶ The tubing may be kinked or pinched in a side rail

▶ The bottle/bag may not be hanging high enough

▶ The tubing may be clamped too tightly

▶ The patient may have shifted position or be lying on the tubing
▶ The tape over the tubing may be too tight
▶ If a volume-control chamber is being used, air may be trapped in the filter, the filter may be wet, or both vents may be closed
▶ If an infusion pump or volume controller is being used, it may have been set up incorrectly or may be malfunctioning
▶ There may be clotting or infiltration at the insertion site (for details, see section B)
▶ The air vent may be occluded (wet)
▶ The roller slide clamp may be closed.

b. Intervention. Examine the entire setup, beginning with the tourniquet (which should be promptly removed) and then proceeding from the bottle/bag down to the puncture site. If you can't find the problem, ask someone more experienced—such as your institution's IV team—for help.

c. Suggestions for prevention
▶ Don't place any constricting device (e.g., restraints) over or directly above an IV site
▶ Check the infusion system regularly.

3. Improper flow rate

a. What may happen. The regulator clamp may have slipped or been tampered with, or it may have been set incorrectly initially.

b. Intervention. Resist the temptation to "catch up" by setting the flow rate faster than the rate prescribed. Also resist the temptation to set the flow rate fast in order to use up the contents of the container. It's better to start a new container and to make sure the clamp is set to permit the correct flow rate.

c. Suggestions for prevention
▶ Calculate the flow rate accurately
▶ Check the system regularly for the prescribed rate of flow.

B. PROBLEMS AT THE INSERTION SITE

1. Extravasation (infiltration)

a. What may happen. The catheter/needle may have been pulled partly or entirely out of the vein, flooding the surrounding tissue with IV solution. The catheter/needle may have perforated the opposite wall of the vein, or the patient's movements may have widened the opening in the vein, causing the contents—blood and IV solution—to leak into the surrounding tissues. Signs of infiltration include these:

▶ Swelling
▶ Pain
▶ Coolness
▶ Slight, or no, blood return.

The consequences of infiltration range from mild and temporary to severe and lasting, and include pain, loss of use of other veins in the infiltrated limb, and permanent damage to nerves. Extravasation of irritating solutions and/or medications may cause necrosis of tissues, and disfigurement or loss of the limb.

b. Intervention
▶ Discontinue the infusion
▶ Using a new venipuncture device, start the infusion at another site
▶ If an irritating solution and/or medication is involved, contact the IV therapy specialist,

the physician, or the pharmacist for possible treatment *before* discontinuing the line

▸ Apply warm, moist compresses for a 20-minute period three or four times a day to ease discomfort at the old site. If the patient complains that warmth doesn't help, try cool compresses.

c. Suggestions for prevention

▸ Use a hand board or arm board to stabilize the catheter/needle when the site is over a joint or the patient is especially active

▸ Palpate the site frequently to check for signs of coolness or swelling of the tissues

▸ Check the site regularly—and especially before infusing medications—for good blood return.

2. Local infection

*a. **What may happen.*** Bacteria may enter the puncture wound by migrating along the skin tract, or contamination may occur due to poor aseptic technique on insertion or poor site maintenance. The site will be sore, with varying degrees of warmth and redness. Foul-smelling, or purulent, drainage may be noted at the site.

b. Intervention

▸ Discontinue the infusion

▸ Culture the catheter, site, and drainage according to your institution's policies and procedures

▸ Clean the site with an antiseptic solution and cover it with a sterile dressing

▸ Restart the IV infusion if necessary—preferably in the opposite limb

▸ Notify the patient's physician

▸ Chart the procedure and your observations in the patient's record.

c. Suggestions for prevention
▸ Maintain aseptic technique when starting an IV infusion
▸ Keep all IV sites clean and dry
▸ Be careful to avoid touch contamination when changing IV tubings, dressings, etc.

3. Clotting

a. What may happen. A fibrin clot may form because the IV solution is flowing at too slow a KVO rate, because the bottle/bag is empty, or because the tubing has become obstructed.

b. Intervention. Try raising the bottle/bag (if it isn't empty), opening the regulator clamp all the way, and "milking" the tubing. If this is unsuccessful, try flushing the tubing (see Chapter 13) through the injection port. Don't force the saline into the tubing, as you may dislodge the clot and push it into the circulation. If these two measures fail, discontinue the infusion and start over at another site, preferably in the opposite limb.

c. Suggestions for prevention
▸ Check the IV frequently to make sure the tubing isn't kinked
▸ Be careful not to allow the IV to run "dry"
▸ Check the flow rate regularly.

4. Phlebitis

a. What may happen. Many things may actually cause phlebitis (the inflammation of a vein). They may be grouped into one of three categories:

▸ Mechanical phlebitis—the catheter/needle movement within the vein may actually irritate and inflame the intima of the vein, causing "mechanical" phlebitis

▸ Chemical phlebitis—various drugs, especially cephalothin (Keflin), gentamicin (Garamycin), minocycline (Minocin), tetracycline (Achromycin), cefamandole (Mandol), potassium chloride, penicillin, and anesthetic agents, have been known to irritate and inflame the vein intima, causing "chemical" phlebitis

▸ Bacterial phlebitis—microorganisms may contaminate the system anywhere along the line. Touch contamination while changing the IV solution or tubing, attaching a piggyback medication, manipulating a stopcock or CVP manometer, injecting into the line, or migration of bacteria along the skin tract into the puncture site may allow for the entrance of bacteria into the body, causing "bacterial" phlebitis.

The severity of phlebitis may be categorized by degrees. Watch for the corresponding signs:

▸ 1°—pain, soreness, or tenderness at the site, without redness

▸ 2°—pain and soreness with redness at, or extending less than 3 inches above, the site

▸ 3°—pain, soreness, and redness extending more than 3 inches above the site, with the presence of a palpable cord in the vein

▸ 4°—pain, soreness, and redness extending more than 3 inches in length above the site and a palpable cord with evidence of exudate at the site.

b. Intervention. If the patient complains of pain while a medication is being infused, try continuing the infusion while applying warm, moist compresses to the limb. If, however, pain continues or increases and/or redness develops, discontinue the infusion and start again elsewhere, if possible in the opposite limb. If you suspect a drug is causing the inflammation, can you administer it in a larger quantity of solution so that it's more dilute? Or can you administer it over a shorter period of time? Carefully watch the old site for signs of infection; culture it according to your institution's policies, particularly if you suspect bacterial phlebitis. Apply warm, moist compresses to the area to help with the healing process. Chart your observations in the patient's record.

c. Suggestions for prevention
- Check the site frequently for signs of soreness or redness
- Infuse the medication at the prescribed rate of flow
- Use the smallest-size catheter/needle that will meet the patient's needs and allow for adequate dilution of the solution and/or medication in the vein
- Dilute irritating medications with as much diluent as possible.

5. Thrombophlebitis

a. What may happen. Thrombophlebitis is a complication of phlebitis. When the wall of the vein becomes irritated and inflamed, blood may collect and form a clot. In addition to pain and redness, there may be considerable swelling around the site. The vein may also feel hard and cordlike, with evidence of warmth and redness and/or a red streak.

b. Intervention. Discontinue the infusion and start a new one in the opposite limb. Apply warm, moist compresses to the old site. Notify a physician. Chart your observations in the patient's record.
NOTE: Suppurative thrombophlebitis—an extremely dangerous systemic complication—is described in section C3. Because this complication can arise after an infusion has been discontinued, it's important to observe the patient carefully.

c. Suggestions for prevention
- Check the site frequently for signs of soreness and/or redness
- Infuse the medication at the prescribed rate of flow
- Use the smallest-size catheter/needle that will meet the patient's needs and allow for adequate dilution in the vein
- Dilute irritating medications with as much diluent as possible
- Develop an atraumatic insertion technique
- Tape the catheter/needle device securely to prevent unnecessary movement of the device in the vein.

6. Hematoma

a. What may happen. Blood may escape from the vein into the surrounding tissues or be infused into the tissues.

b. Intervention
- If, during a transfusion, the blood is infused into the tissues, discontinue the infusion. Using a new venipuncture device, start the

transfusion at another site, preferably in the opposite limb

▸ If blood has escaped into the surrounding tissues because of a through-and-through penetration of the vein, remove the catheter/needle device and apply digital pressure to the site until the bleeding stops; if the bleeding appears to be severe and/or prolonged, cool compresses or an ice pack may be applied to the area

▸ Once the possibility of continued bleeding into the tissues has ceased, warm, moist compresses may be applied to the limb to enhance the healing process.

c. Suggestions for prevention

▸ Check to be sure you have a patent IV line *before* initiating a blood transfusion

▸ Check the patient's site frequently during a transfusion

▸ Develop a smooth insertion technique

▸ When initiating a venipuncture, vary the angle of entry according to the individual needs of the patient, to prevent through-and-through penetration of the vein

▸ Use a direct venipuncture approach when initiating a venipuncture on a patient with "fragile" veins.

C. SYSTEMIC PROBLEMS

1. Side effects, drug interactions, and adverse or allergic reactions

a. What may happen. The interaction or incompatibility of certain drugs, or the patient's sensitivity to a specific solution or medication may produce signs of adverse or allergic reactions. Some of these signs may include, but are not limited to:

► GI disturbances
► Central nervous system (CNS) depression
► Respiratory symptoms
► Anaphylaxis
► Rash/pruritus.

These complications depend on the drug or drugs being given, on the dose and route of each, and on the individual patient. Obviously this book can't cover such a large topic. You should, however, be aware of the common side effects, interactions, and adverse reactions that can occur with drugs that are given intravenously.

b. Intervention

► Slow the infusion to a KVO rate (if the symptoms are mild or questionable), or discontinue the infusion but keep the line open with 0.9% NaCl (NSS)
► Notify the patient's physician
► Chart your observations.

c. Suggestions for prevention

► Check the patient's history of allergies before beginning an infusion
► Observe the patient frequently
► Administer the solution and/or medication according to the pharmacist's and the manufacturer's recommendations.

2. Septicemia

a. What may happen. Bacteria or fungi may be introduced into an IV line at any point where one part is connected to another, particularly where the connection is performed manually. Poor design of IV equipment and improper manufacturing and storage have also been implicated in outbreaks of septicemia. Watch for these signs:

- Fever and/or chills
- Cold sweats
- Drop in blood pressure
- Nausea, vomiting, or diarrhea
- Increase in pulse rate.

b. Intervention. Notify the physician. Consider other possible sites of origin for the septicemia (respiratory infection, urinary tract infection, wound infection, etc.) and culture any suspected sites. If no other sources of infection can be found, the IV system must be considered as the possible source—with or without signs of local infection. The IV site, tubing, bottle/bag, and any attachments should be cultured in accordance with your institution's policies, as outlined in Chapter 19. If the patient must continue to receive infusion therapy, another line may be started if necessary, but preferably in the opposite limb. Chart the procedure and your observations in the patient's record.

c. Suggestions for prevention

- Always maintain aseptic technique
- Be careful not to contaminate the system when changing solutions, tubings, and dressings
- Keep all IV sites clean, dry, and covered with an antibacterial ointment/solution and sterile dressing.

3. Suppurative thrombophlebitis

a. What may happen. The chain of events leading to this potentially fatal complication might start with irritation of the venous wall. Organisms enter the vein via contaminated IV solution, tubing, or insertion site. These organisms infect the irritated venous wall and a pocket of pus forms. This purulent thrombus then embolizes, releasing huge numbers of infective organisms into the patient's circulation and producing overwhelming sepsis.

b. Intervention. Unfortunately, signs of severe septicemia may be the first clinical warning of suppurative thrombophlebitis. Notify a physician and discontinue the infusion. The site, tubing, bottle/bag, and any attachments should be cultured in accordance with your institution's policies, as outlined in Chapter 19. Another line may be started, if necessary, in the opposite limb. Chart the procedure and your observations in the patient's record.

c. Suggestions for prevention. They are the same as those for septicemia.

4. Air embolism

a. What may happen. Air inadvertently introduced into the IV line may enter a vein. As little as 50 to 100 ml of air can cause an embolism in an adult; less will do so in a small child. There is an even greater possibility that an air embolism will occur when dealing with a central line than when dealing with a peripheral line. An air embolism produces these symptoms:

▶ Drop in blood pressure
▶ Rapid, thready pulse
▶ Crushing chest pain

▶ Difficulty breathing, progressing to failure
▶ Cyanosis.

b. Intervention
▶ Turn the patient on his or her left side and lower the head of the bed (Trendelenburg position)
▶ Try to determine the source of the air (e.g., disconnected line)
▶ Give the patient oxygen (2 to 3 liters)
▶ Notify the physician
▶ Chart what you did and your observations in the patient's record.

c. Suggestions for prevention
▶ Make sure all connections on the IV line are securely fastened
▶ Purge all air from the tubing before connecting the tubing to the patient
▶ Change all tubings quickly, especially on central lines. You may have the patient forcibly exhale (Valsalva maneuver) when changing tubing on a central line.

5. Catheter embolism
This is a greater possibility when inserting a CTN device than when using a CON device.

a. What may happen.
A piece of catheter may be severed and may enter the circulatory system.

b. Intervention
▶ Discontinue the IV infusion
▶ Apply a tourniquet to the patient's limb above the insertion site. Apply the tourniquet so that it is tight enough to restrict venous flow but not arterial flow

- ▶ Notify the physician and have the patient X-rayed to locate the severed catheter
- ▶ Chart what you did and your observations in the patient's record.

c. Suggestions for prevention
- ▶ Never reinsert the needle/stylet in the catheter once it has been withdrawn
- ▶ Take special care when you withdraw a CTN device
- ▶ When using scissors to remove an IV dressing, be extremely careful that the catheter isn't accidentally cut.

6. Circulatory overload

a. What may happen.
The patient may receive too much fluid for the circulatory system to handle. Circulatory overload produces these symptoms:

- ▶ Increase in blood pressure
- ▶ Distended veins in the neck, face, and arms
- ▶ Respirations become shallow and rapid (dyspnea)
- ▶ Rales may be detected
- ▶ Frothy sputum
- ▶ Productive cough.

b. Intervention
- ▶ Slow the infusion to a KVO rate
- ▶ Elevate the head of the bed
- ▶ Apply oxygen (2 to 3 liters), provided it is not contraindicated
- ▶ Notify the patient's physician
- ▶ Chart what you did and your observations in the patient's record.

c. Suggestions for prevention

- ▶ Monitor the patient's vital signs and intake and output carefully
- ▶ Check the infusion flow rate regularly and notify the physician if it appears to be more than the patient can tolerate
- ▶ Be aware of the patient's cardiovascular status and history before beginning the infusion.

CHAPTER **16**

CHAPTER

Blood transfusions

Whole blood isn't often administered. However, since administration of whole blood and certain of its constituents—particularly packed red cells—creates unique problems, it's important to learn the rules and considerations that govern blood transfusions.

A. TERMINOLOGY

▶ *Agglutination*: The clumping of red cells by the formation of antibody bridges between antigens on different cells

▶ *Antibody*: Protein in plasma that may react with a specific antigen

▶ *Antigen*: A substance that has the ability to evoke an immune response when injected into an individual to whom it is foreign

▶ *Bacteriolysin*: An antibody produced within the body that is capable of bringing about the dissolution or lysis of bacteria

▶ *HLA*: Human leukocyte antigen
▶ *Immunoglobulins*: Proteins with known antibody activity
▶ *Rh (Rhesus)*: The presence or absence of red blood cell D antigen
▶ *Titer*: The amount of antibody in a serum.

B. BLOOD COMPONENTS

1. Plasma
▶ Water
▶ Gases
▶ Protein (albumin, globulins, fibrinogen)
▶ Salts (chlorides, bicarbonates, sulfates, phosphates)
▶ Protective substances (antibodies, bacteriolysins)
▶ Waste (urea, creatinine).

2. Cells
▶ Red blood cells—erythrocytes
▶ White blood cells—leukocytes (basophils, eosinophils, neutrophils, lymphocytes, monocytes)
▶ Platelets.

C. COMPATIBILITY

Never give whole blood or packed red cells unless you're certain of donor-recipient compatibility, except in an extreme emergency on the orders of a physician. Type O blood may be administered in controlled situations (e.g., ER, OR, trauma unit) when dealing with life-and-death situations. Transfusion of a wrong blood type is prevented by crossmatching the donor's blood with the recipient's blood prior to initiation of the transfusion. Blood types are differentiated by their antigen and antibody content (see Table 16-1).

Table 16-1

Antigen and antibody content of various blood types

Blood type	Antigen type (found in RBCs)	Antibody type (found in plasma)
A	A	Anti-B
B	B	Anti-A
AB	A and B	None
O	None	Anti-A and anti-B

1. Requirements for different components

Blood is frequently utilized in component parts. Various components are indicated in specific circumstances. Not all of these components require typing and crossmatching. For those that do, however, the compatibility requirement is absolute, except as noted above. Table 16-2 is a guide to the infusion of blood and its various components.

2. Safety

You may have the right blood, but the wrong recipient. A mistake like that could have disastrous—even fatal—results. Thus, the importance of safety cannot be overstressed. To help prevent mistakes, the following steps are strongly recommended:

▶ Check the physician's order for the transfusion
▶ If the patient is conscious, ask his/her name

Table 16-2

Component therapy

Product	Indications for use	Average infusion time	Cross-matching
Whole blood	Increase blood volume. ▲ Hemorrhage ▲ Trauma.	2-4 hr	ABO and Rh
Packed red blood cells	Increase red cell mass. ▲ Anemia.	2-3 hr	ABO and Rh
Washed red blood cells	Increase red cell mass; prevent tissue antigen formation. ▲ Immunosuppressed patients ▲ Patients with previous transfusion reactions.	1-2 hr	ABO and Rh
White blood cells (leukophoresis)	Agranulocytosis.	60-90 min	ABO and HLA (preferably leukocyte group A antigen)

Fresh frozen plasma (FFP); 30-45 min for thawing	Coagulation disorders; hypovolemia. ▲ Burn patients.	15-45 min	None
Platelets	Thrombocytopenia. ▲ Leukemia patients ▲ Patients receiving massive transfusions.	30-45 min for drip infusion; 5-10 min for IV push	ABO
Cryoprecipitate (factor VIII)	Bleeding disorder due to lack of factor VIII; fibrinogen deficiency. ▲ Hemophilia ▲ Von Willebrand's disease.	15-30 min for drip infusion; 10-15 min for IV push	ABO
Factor II, VII, IX, X complex	Bleeding disorder due to lack of these factors. ▲ Christmas disease.	15-30 min	None
Albumin, 5% or 25%	Blood volume expansion; replacement of protein. ▲ Burn patients ▲ Hypoproteinemia.	30-60 min	None
Plasma protein fraction	Blood volume expansion; replacement of protein. ▲ Hypovolemia ▲ Hypoproteinemia.	30-60 min	None

► Check the patient's name, birth date, and hospital identification number on the patient's ID bracelet with the label on the blood product
► Have a second person recheck the above information with you
► Take the patient's vital signs; if they are not within normal limits for that patient, notify the physician before initiating the transfusion
► Be sure you have a patent line with an appropriate catheter/needle device. Normal (0.9%) saline is the *only* acceptable solution that may immediately precede or flush a blood infusion line
► Record the procedure, and the number of the blood product infusing, in the patient's record
► Monitor the patient's vital signs throughout the infusion (q 15 min × 2, then q 30 min until the procedure is finished).

D. EQUIPMENT FOR ADMINISTERING WHOLE BLOOD, PACKED RED CELLS, AND WASHED RED CELLS

1. Catheter/needle for venipuncture

a. Whole blood and washed red cells. Use an 18-, 20-, or 22-gauge catheter: the largest size permitted by the patient's venous system and physical condition. For transfusion through a scalp vein, needles as small as 25 gauge may be used.

b. Packed red cells. An 18-gauge catheter is best, but you may use a 20-gauge device for venipuncture if necessary.

2. Normal (0.9%) saline

In some institutions, it's customary to precede and follow transfusions of whole blood or blood components with normal saline. If normal saline isn't already running, you may use a 250- or 500-ml bottle of normal saline solution.

3. Straight-line blood set

This may be either a primary or secondary set. The drip chamber contains a filter, so you don't have to add a filter to the line. Use a large (16- or 18-gauge) needle to infuse the blood or packed cells into the primary line if the blood set is a secondary set. If the primary solution is not normal saline, you'll have to replace it with normal saline. A straight-line set is also used for administering plasma, white cells, plasma protein fraction, and factors II, VII, IX, and X complex. The blood set should be changed after the infusion of two units.

4. Y blood set

A Y set may also be either a primary or secondary set. It's especially useful when the primary solution is not normal saline, as you don't have to replace the primary solution. A Y set is advantageous for transfusion of packed red cells because it enables you to dilute the viscous cells with saline if necessary. Like a straight-line set, a Y set contains a filter in the drip chamber (see Figure 16-1). Attach the saline to one arm of the Y set and the unit of blood to the other. To keep blood from backing up into the primary line, if you are piggybacking the Y blood set into the primary set, close the clamp on the primary set. The Y set should be changed after the infusion of two units of blood.

5. Microaggregate recipient set and filters

   a. A microaggregate recipient set is used to transfuse large amounts—more than three units—of blood for immunosuppressed patients or for those with potential febrile leukocyte reactions. The special filter

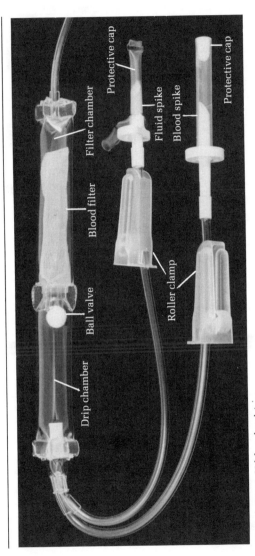

Figure 16-1 Y blood tubing

prevents lysed cells from reaching the patient's circulation, and the large tubing permits rapid administration. A microaggregate set may be used as a primary or secondary set.

b. Microaggregate add-on filters are added to straight IV tubing when three or more units of blood are to be infused over a short period of time. They function exactly the same way as microaggregate recipient sets except that the filter is separate and must be added to the IV tubing. Frequently used microaggregate filters are Bentley, Pall, Fenwal, and Swank.

6. Blood warmers

Never give large amounts of cold blood rapidly; that's likely to cause venous spasms and/or shock. Blood warmers should be used for patients receiving multiple units of blood, for those receiving blood through a central line, and for those who have cold agglutinins present in their blood.

a. Coil type. Prime the coil, then close all clamps. Immerse the filled coil in water warmed to 99°F (37.6°C), taking care to keep both adapters dry.

b. Electric type. After putting the blood-warming bag in the warmer and closing the door, let the warmer heat to 99°F. Prime the line with saline and start the transfusion according to the manufacturer's directions.

7. Transfusion pumps

Pumps are used to administer large amounts of blood quickly. They are not used routinely, and should be operated only by qualified personnel. Both types described here are operated by manual pressure. If you're using a very small catheter/needle, pumping can mechanically lyse red cells.

a. Built-in type. This is a complete primary or secondary administration set, primed like any other. Make sure the pump chamber is completely filled before you squeeze it.

b. Slip-on type. This pump may be used with a straight-line or Y-type set. After priming the set, slip the pump bag over the blood bag and hang both together. Open the screw clamp and squeeze the bulb until the gauge shows the desired pressure reading. Don't make the pressure so great that the needle on the pressure gauge goes into the red (danger) area.

E. EQUIPMENT FOR ADMINISTERING CRYOPRECIPITATE AND PLATELETS

1. Catheter/needle for venipuncture
An 18-gauge catheter is best, but a 20-gauge device may be used for venipuncture if necessary.

2. Component syringe set
A component syringe set is a secondary set. It permits rapid infusion of platelets—an important feature, since slow administration is likely to clog the primary line. The spiked (clamped) arm of this Y-shaped set is attached to the component bag; the other arm is connected to a 50- or 60-ml syringe. With the lower clamp closed, fill the syringe. Then close the upper clamp, open the lower one, and administer the component at the prescribed rate by IV push.

3. Component drip set
A component drip set can be used as either a secondary or a primary set.

F. CARE AND HANDLING OF BLOOD

1. Contamination
Blood and blood components are precious.
They're also especially fertile breeding grounds for microorganisms. Take extra care to avoid inadvertent contamination when performing a transfusion.

2. Mixing whole blood
Red cells tend to settle and plasma tends to rise, so mix whole blood thoroughly. Avoid excessive agitation, though, as it may destroy cells. Gently rock the bag during transfusion to keep the red cells and plasma mixed.

3. Rate of administration
Federal regulations require that whole blood or packed red cells be transfused at rates no slower than one unit in four hours. Washed, packed, or fresh frozen red cells may be infused for between one and two hours, but no longer than four hours. Transfusions faster than one unit per hour should only be done if the patient's condition can tolerate it and in extreme emergencies under carefully controlled conditions.

G. MONITORING TRANSFUSIONS

Transfusion reactions may occur during, immediately after, or up to 96 hours following the transfusion.

1. Vital signs
Record vital signs just before and after each transfusion. During a transfusion, record vital signs every 15 minutes for the first half hour, and then every half hour until the transfusion is completed, or according to your institution's policy.

2. Hemolytic reactions

a. Cause. Hemolytic reactions are due to separation of hemoglobin from either the recipient's or the donor's red cells during or following a transfusion. Hemolysis may be caused by any of several factors:

- ▶ Blood group incompatibility
- ▶ Rh incompatibility
- ▶ Injection of water or nonisotonic solutions.

b. Severity. The severity of a hemolytic reaction depends on:

- ▶ The degree of ABO or Rh incompatibility
- ▶ The amount of blood administered
- ▶ The rate of administration
- ▶ The condition of the patient's liver, kidneys, and heart
- ▶ The temperature of the blood.

c. Symptoms. If the patient complains of any of these symptoms, first try to rule out other causes, such as a history of emphysema, recovery from surgery under a general anesthetic, or the temperature of the room.

- ▶ Generalized tingling sensation
- ▶ Increased discomfort or anxiety
- ▶ Difficulty breathing
- ▶ Precordial pressure
- ▶ Bursting sensation in the head that isn't due to anesthesia—a frequent cause of headache
- ▶ Flushed face
- ▶ Temperature elevation of more than 2°F
- ▶ Chills not due to hypothermia caused by anesthesia

▸ Severe pain in the neck, chest, or lumbar area that isn't due to positioning during surgery or to preexisting conditions.

d. Intervention

▸ Check once more the patient's ID and blood numbers
▸ Clamp off the blood line, if it's still running, and administer normal saline
▸ Notify the physician and the laboratory
▸ Obtain required blood and urine samples
▸ Wait for the results of laboratory tests: If positive, disconnect the transfusion set, send it and the remaining blood to the lab, and notify the physician; if negative, slowly restart the transfusion and carefully observe the patient.

e. Prevention

▸ Double-check the patient's name, identification number, and blood type before initiating the transfusion
▸ Monitor the patient closely during the transfusion, especially during the first 30 minutes.

3. Pyrogenic reactions

a. Cause. Pyrogenic reactions following transfusions are systemic reactions due to leukocyte agglutination or the presence of bacterial lipopolysaccharides.

b. Symptoms. First rule out other causes for the following symptoms:

▸ Chills
▸ Temperature elevation of more than 2°F
▸ Pain in the extremities or back.

c. Intervention. Take the same steps as outlined for hemolytic reactions.

d. Prevention
- An antipyretic medication may be administered prior to initiating the transfusion
- If the patient has had a previous reaction, washed or fresh frozen packed red cells should be used
- Keep the patient covered and warm during the transfusion
- Use a microaggregate blood filter.

4. Allergic reactions

a. Cause. Allergic reactions are caused by hypersensitivity to some component of the donor's blood.

b. Symptoms. First rule out other causes for the following symptoms:
- Urticaria and pruritus
- Edema
- Dizziness and/or headache
- Nausea
- Chills (may be accompanied by a temperature elevation)
- Wheezing or dyspnea
- Lumbar pain.

c. Intervention. Take the same steps as outlined for hemolytic reactions.

d. Prevention
- If the patient has had a previous reaction, washed or fresh frozen packed red cells should be used
- An antihistamine (e.g., Benadryl) may be ordered prior to initiating the transfusion

▶ Monitor the patient closely during the transfusion, especially during the first 30 minutes.

5. Circulatory overload

a. Cause. Circulatory overload may occur in the presence of heart disease with long-standing anemia. Circulatory overload may also occur when the cardiac musculature and reserve are deficient.

b. Symptoms. First rule out other causes for the following symptoms:

▶ Pulmonary congestion
▶ Signs of right-sided heart failure
▶ Dilated neck and arm veins
▶ Moist rales
▶ Flushed feeling
▶ Edema.

c. Intervention. Take the same steps as outlined for hemolytic reactions.

d. Prevention

▶ Use packed or washed red cells when the patient's cardiovascular system may be compromised
▶ Infuse the blood slowly
▶ Keep the patient warm and in a Fowler's position
▶ A diuretic may be ordered prior to initiating the transfusion
▶ Monitor the patient closely during the transfusion.

6. Septicemia

a. Cause. Septicemia may be caused by infusion of contaminated blood or blood products, or by the presence of microorganisms somewhere within the transfusion line. Chapter 15 details the symptoms of septicemia.

b. Intervention

▶ Check once again the patient's ID and blood numbers
▶ Clamp off the blood line, if it's still running, and administer normal saline
▶ Notify the physician
▶ Obtain required blood and urine samples
▶ Culture the puncture site, tubing, and bag in accordance with your institution's policy (see Chapter 19)
▶ Wait for the results of laboratory tests: If positive, disconnect the transfusion set, send it and the remaining blood to the lab, and notify the physician; if negative, slowly restart the transfusion and carefully observe the patient.

c. Prevention

▶ Use strict aseptic technique when handling blood and blood products
▶ Avoid touch contamination of the infusion line
▶ Infuse the blood within the prescribed time
▶ Change the blood tubing after every one to two units.

CHAPTER 17

Fluids and electrolytes

We infuse many solutions and medications into our patients intravenously. These substances contain a variety of ingredients (electrolytes, vitamins, medications, etc.) and place a variety of demands on the body to adjust. Different disease processes, surgical procedures, and changes in physiology also produce a number of requirements and adjustments for the body to meet. If we are to be successful in restoring and maintaining the body in a state of homeostasis, and if we are to help our patients realize their optimal level of health and functioning, we must have a basic understanding of fluids and electrolytes, and learn to apply those principles in caring for our patients—particularly those requiring intravenous therapy.

A. TERMINOLOGY

▸ *Anions:* Negatively charged ions
▸ *Cations:* Positively charged ions

- *Colloids:* Substances that do not dissolve in solution but form a gelatin-like substance
- *Crenation:* An alteration of the external wall of a red blood cell due to a change in the internal fluid content
- *Crystalloids:* Substances that completely dissolve to form a clear solution
- *Diffusion:* Movement of solute molecules (gas, liquid, or solid) across a selectively permeable membrane from an area of high concentration to one of lower concentration
- *Electrolytes:* Electrically charged particles (ions)
- *Extracellular:* Outside the cell
- *Filtration:* The transfer of water and dissolved substances through a selectively permeable membrane from an area of high concentration to one of low concentration, based on hydrostatic pressure (mm Hg)—diffusion under pressure
- *Hemolysis:* Movement of water from extracellular to intracellular space, which causes the red blood cell to swell and rupture
- *Hypertonic:* Having a higher osmotic pressure than a compared solution
- *Hypotonic:* Having a lower osmotic pressure than a compared solution
- *Intracellular:* Inside the cell
- *Isotonic:* A solution having a comparable concentration of solute particles that will exert an equivalent amount of osmotic pressure as that solution with which it is being compared
- *Milliequivalent (mEq):* Measures the concentration of electrolytes in solution. Their chemical combining power is based on the number of available ionic charges in the solution
- *Milliosmole (mOsm):* Measurement of osmotic activity in a given solution. The normal osmolality of body fluids is 280 to 294 mOsm/kg

► *Osmosis:* Movement of water across a semipermeable membrane from the area of lower concentration to the area of higher concentration, thus tending to equalize the concentration of the two solutions

► *Osmotic pressure:* The pressure that develops when two solutions of different concentrations are separated by a semipermeable membrane. Osmotic pressure varies with the concentration of the solution and with temperature variations

► *Solutes:* Particles that are suspended or dissolved in a solvent

► *Solution:* Made up of a solvent and solutes

► *Solvent:* A liquid

► *Tonicity:* The concentration of dissolved particles in solution as compared with plasma.

B. BODY FLUIDS

1. Water (H_2O)

a. Amount. The amount of water contained in the body is dependent on:

► Age
► Weight
► Sex.

b. Body weight. The percentage of body weight accounted for by water is:

► Average male—60%
► Average female—54%
► Average infant—80%.

2. Compartments

a. Intracellular. This compartment accounts for approximately 40% of body weight.

b. Extracellular

► Interstitial (surrounds the cell)—accounts for approximately 15% of body weight

► Intravascular (within the blood vessels)—accounts for approximately 5% of body weight.

3. Electrolytes

In order to achieve chemical balance, the total number of positive charges must equal the total number of negative charges within each fluid compartment of the body.

► Principal extracellular electrolytes: Na^+, Ca^{2+}, Cl^-, HCO_3^-

► Principal intracellular electrolytes: K^+, Mg^{2+}, PO_4^{3-}.

See section C below for a discussion of individual electrolytes.

4. Nonelectrolytes

a. Dextrose (D-Glucose)

► Normal serum level: 80 to 120 mg/dl
► Function: supplies necessary calories for energy (spares protein); converted to glycogen by the liver (improves hepatic function); daily requirement is approximately 100 grams per day.

b. Urea nitrogen

► Normal serum level: 10 to 20 mg/dl.

c. Creatinine

► Normal serum level: 1 to 1.5 mg/dl.

C. ELECTROLYTES

1. Sodium (Na^+)

Sodium is the principal extracellular cation.

► Normal serum level: 135 to 145 mEq/L
► Function: regulates osmotic pressure of extracellular fluid and water balance within the

body; also assists in the transmission of nerve impulses and influences the body's acid-base balance.

a. Hyponatremia
- Some causes: CHF; impaired renal function; cirrhosis; prolonged fever; diarrhea, vomiting, or gastric suctioning; burns; adrenal insufficiency; increased diaphoresis (a total day's sodium may be lost with 6 to 8 hours of diaphoresis)
- Signs and symptoms: muscle weakness; headache; decreased skin turgor; tremors and/or convulsions; serum sodium <135 mEq/L.

b. Hypernatremia
- Some causes: inadequate water intake; excess sodium intake; excessive water losses as in prolonged diarrhea; vomiting; polyuria; diabetes mellitus
- Signs and symptoms: thirst; dry, sticky membranes; fever; flushed skin; oliguria; serum sodium >145 mEq/L.

2. Potassium (K^+)
Potassium is the principal intracellular cation.

- Normal serum level: 3.5 to 5.3 mEq/L
- Function: regulates cellular osmotic pressure; activates enzymes; regulates acid-base balance; assists with nerve impulse transmission in nerves and muscles.

a. Hypokalemia
- Some causes: renal dysfunction; CHF; excessive use of diuretics; prolonged gastric suctioning; vomiting; diaphoresis or diarrhea; adrenal disorders; liver disease; starvation; ulcerative colitis; polyuria

▶ Signs and symptoms: decreased gastrointestinal, skeletal, and cardiac muscle function; decreased reflexes; muscular irritability or weakness; rapid, weak, and irregular pulse; decreased blood pressure; nausea and vomiting; paralytic ileus; ECG changes; postural hypotension.

b. Hyperkalemia

▶ Some causes: renal failure; massive cell damage, as in trauma, burns, major surgery, and myocardial infarction

▶ Signs and symptoms: muscle weakness; nausea; diarrhea; muscle irritability; oliguria; ECG changes.

3. Calcium (Ca^{2+})

▶ Normal serum level: 8.5 to 10.5 mg/dl

▶ Function: important in formation and function of bones and teeth; aids in blood clotting; regulates neuromuscular excitability; assists in transfer of Na^+ across semipermeable membrane.

u. Hypocalcemia

▶ Some causes: hypoparathyroidism; vitamin D or magnesium deficiency; pancreatitis; post-op thyroid or parathyroid patients; diarrhea; extensive infections; patients on prolonged TPN or dialysis; burns

▶ Signs and symptoms: muscle twitching and cramps; perioral paresthesias; carpopedal spasms; tetany; convulsions.

b. Hypercalcemia

▶ Some causes: hyperparathyroidism; overdose of vitamin D or antacids; skeletal diseases; carcinomas (such as parathyroid adenoma and multiple myeloma)

▸ Signs and symptoms: lethargy; anorexia; nausea; vomiting; constipation; dehydration; cardiac arrhythmias; coma.

4. Magnesium (Mg^{2+})

▸ Normal serum level: 1.5 to 2.5 mEq/L
▸ Function: controls action of enzymes; assists in metabolism of proteins and carbohydrates; aids in controlling neuromuscular irritability; facilitates transportation of Na^+ and K^+ across cell membranes.

a. Hypomagnesemia. This condition usually coexists with low Ca^{2+} and K^+ levels.

▸ Some causes: impaired gastrointestinal absorption; diarrhea; inadequate diet; hyperparathyroidism; excessive use of diuretics; prolonged vomiting or nasogastric suctioning; renal dysfunction; chronic alcoholism
▸ Signs and symptoms: cardiac arrhythmias; muscle weakness; seizures; tremors; tetany; cramps in the lower extremities; insomnia; disorientation.

b. Hypermagnesemia

▸ Some causes: renal failure; excessive use of antacids
▸ Signs and symptoms: hypotension; flushing; sweating; slow, weak pulse; lethargy; decreased respirations; muscle weakness; decreased reflexes; coma; bradycardia; heart block; cardiac arrest.

5. Chloride (Cl^-)

▸ Normal serum level: 95 to 109 mEq/L
▸ Function: competes with bicarbonate for combination with Na^+ ions; assists in maintaining acid-base balance.

a. Hypochloremia

▸ Some causes: prolonged nasogastric suctioning; excessive use of diuretics; prolonged diaphoresis, gastrointestinal suctioning; diabetic ketosis; CHF; renal failure; low-salt diet; metabolic alkalosis

▸ Signs and symptoms: increased muscle excitability; tetany; decreased respirations.

b. Hyperchloremia

▸ Some causes: dehydration; hyperparathyroidism; metabolic acidosis; respiratory alkalosis

▸ Signs and symptoms: stupor; deep, rapid breathing; coma; muscle weakness.

6. Phosphate (PO_4^{3-})

▸ Normal serum level: 1.7 to 2.3 mEq/L

▸ Function: assists with glucose metabolism in red cells; essential for ATP (adenosine triphosphate) formation; acts as a check and balance for Ca^{2+} (inverse relationship with calcium).

a. Hypophosphatemia

▸ Some causes: hyperparathyroidism; rickets; osteomalacia; abnormalities of the renal tubules

▸ Signs and symptoms: circumoral and peripheral paresthesia; lethargy; speech defects (stuttering or stammering).

b. Hyperphosphatemia

▸ Some causes: excessive growth hormone (acromegaly); hypoparathyroidism or pseudohypoparathyroidism; renal insufficiency or acute failure; hypervitaminosis D

▸ Signs and symptoms: usually none.

7. Bicarbonate (HCO_3^-)
▶ Normal serum level: 24 to 32 mEq/L
▶ Function: chief buffer in maintaining acid-base balance (a deficit will cause metabolic acidosis and an overabundance will result in metabolic alkalosis).

8. Proteinate
a. Albumin
▶ Normal serum level: 3.5 to 5.5 g/dl
▶ Function: assists with cell repair; healing of wounds; synthesis of vitamins and enzymes; moving substances from the interstitial fluid into the vascular system; maintaining colloidal osmotic pressure.

b. Globulin
▶ Normal serum level: 1.5 to 3 g/dl
▶ Function: same as for albumin.

9. Sulfate (SO_4^{2-})
▶ Normal serum level: 0.5 to 1.5 mg/dl
▶ Function: basic material of proteins; assists in maintaining acid-base balance.

10. Carbonic acid
Carbonic acid may act as a cation or an anion.

▶ Function: acts as a buffer in maintaining balance between the number of cations and anions in the body.

11. Trace elements
a. Cobalt
▶ Function: the principal constituent of vitamin B_{12}.

b. Copper
▶ Function: essential in preventing anemia.

c. Iodine
▶ Function: essential for thyroid function.
d. Zinc
▶ Function: essential for wound healing and enzyme activity.
e. Manganese
▶ Function: essential for skeletal growth, and Ca^{2+} and phosphorus metabolism.

D. VITAMINS

Vitamins are necessary for the utilization of nutrients and for physiological functions.

1. B and C
▶ Water soluble
▶ Important in metabolism of carbohydrates; promote healing; help maintain gastrointestinal function.

2. A, D, E, and K
▶ Fat soluble
▶ Important in bone formation, calcium and phosphorus absorption, and prothrombin formation
▶ Overingestion may cause hypervitaminosis.

E. ACID-BASE BALANCE

The acid-base balance depends on the hydrogen ion concentration.

1. Normal pH of blood
The normal range of pH in extracellular fluid is 7.35 to 7.45 (extreme limits compatible with life are 6.9 to 7.8).

2. Regulatory mechanisms

The body attempts to maintain its fluid and electrolyte balance through utilization of:

▶ Circulatory (cardiovascular) buffer system
▶ Respiratory system (lungs)
▶ Renal system (kidneys)
▶ Endocrine system (posterior pituitary, parathyroids, adrenals).

F. MONITORING PARAMETERS

A patient's fluid and electrolyte status requires careful monitoring.

1. Clinical monitoring measures

a. Central venous pressure

b. Pulse. Monitoring includes both quality and rate.

c. Venous fill of peripheral veins. The normal venous fill is 3 to 5 seconds.

d. Weight. A 5% change in body weight indicates a serious shift; 1 kilogram of body weight (2.2 pounds) reflects 1 liter of body fluid.

e. Thirst. This occurs with loss of 1 liter of body fluid.

f. I&O (intake and output). Output should equal 30 to 50 ml/hr.

g. Skin turgor

h. Edema

▶ Generalized (e.g., CHF)
▶ Localized (e.g., ascites)
▶ Peripheral.

2. **Laboratory monitoring measures**
   a. Electrolyte studies
   b. Blood cell count and hematocrit. These detect hemoconcentration or hemodilution.
   c. BUN
   d. Serum protein measurement with albumin-globulin ratio

G. FLUID THERAPY

1. Quality of solution
Before initiating infusion, check solution for:

▸ Valid expiration date
▸ Clarity (no particles or cloudiness).

2. Tonicity of solution
Tonicity affects fluid and electrolyte balance.

   a. Hypertonic fluids. Hypertonic fluids (e.g., 3% or 5% NaCl or 10%, 20%, 50% dextrose) increase the osmotic pressure of the blood plasma and draw fluid out of the cells, causing shrinkage of the red blood cells—crenation— if infused over a long period of time* (see Figure 17-1). Such fluids:

   ▸ Should be infused through large (central) veins to allow for rapid dilution
   ▸ May cause osmotic diuresis and cellular dehydration if infused too rapidly or for an extended period of time.

   b. Hypotonic fluids. Hypotonic fluids (e.g., 2.5% dextrose, 0.2% and 0.45% NaCl) decrease the osmotic pressure of the blood plasma and draw fluid into the cells, resulting

---

*New theory may disagree with this concept.

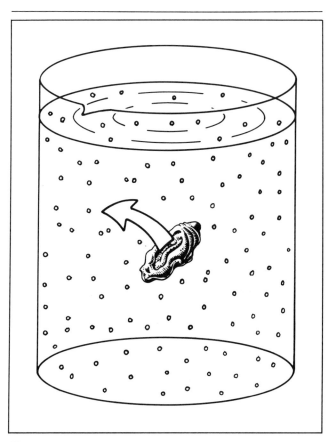

Figure 17-1 Crenation

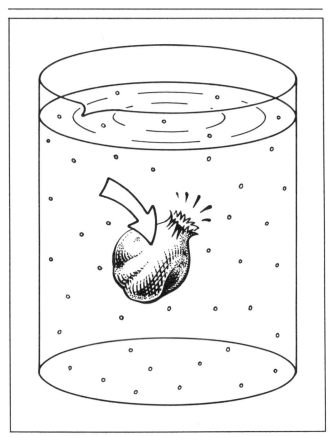

Figure 17-2 Hemolysis

in rupture of the red blood cells—
hemolysis—if infused over a long period of
time (see Figure 17-2). Such fluids:

▶ May be infused through peripheral veins
▶ May produce water intoxication and
  cerebral edema if infused for an extended
  period of time.

c. Isotonic fluids. Isotonic fluids (e.g., 5%
dextrose, 0.9% NaCl, lactated Ringer's)
maintain the osmotic pressure of the blood
plasma and increase the extracellular fluid
volume. Such fluids:

▶ May be infused through peripheral veins
▶ May result in circulatory overload if
  infused over a prolonged period of time or
  too rapidly.

3. Normal maintenance

a. Water

▶ Individual requirements based on age,
  weight, and sex
▶ Insensible losses equal approximately
  1,000 to 1,500 ml per day
▶ Additional losses through urine, feces, and
  vomitus
▶ Essential for all body functions—primary
  constituent of all body fluids
▶ Hypotonic—must be combined with NaCl
  or dextrose to be given intravenously.

b. Glucose

▶ Normal serum level: 80 to 120 mg/dl;
  maintained by action of insulin produced
  by the islets of Langerhans of the pancreas
▶ Daily requirement for the average adult:
  100 grams per day

▸ Supplies necessary calories for energy—spares body protein

▸ Most important carbohydrate in body metabolism—excess glucose is converted to glycogen by the liver.

c. Protein. Amino acids represent the basic structure of proteins.

▸ Daily requirement based on age, weight, daily activities, and state of health: average adult—1 gram per kilogram of body weight per day; average child—2 to 2.2 grams per kilogram of body weight per day

▸ Essential for growth, maintenance, and repair of body tissues

▸ Major source of heat and energy for the body.

d. Fats

▸ Daily requirement for the average adult: 50 to 130 grams per day (restricted intake for patients with hepatitis or those on low-caloric diets)

▸ Important source of energy—spares body protein

▸ Provides essential fatty acids necessary for normal growth and development

▸ Serves as vehicle for absorption of fat-soluble vitamins.

4. Replacement of losses

a. Maintain intake and output record. Adequate kidney function is critical when infusing large amounts of fluids and electrolytes.

b. Monitor patient. The body's need for fluid and electrolyte replacement increases when:

▸ The patient is febrile

▸ The patient is diaphoretic

▶ Cell trauma occurs (due to injury, surgery)
▶ Respirations are increased.

c. Verify type. Type of replacement depends
on type of loss.

H. TYPES OF FLUID

We cannot possibly cover all the types of intravenous
fluid available on the market, but the following are
commonly used solutions.

1. Dextrose in water

a. 5% *(isotonic)*
▶ Daily adult requirement: 1,500 to 2,500 ml
per day
▶ Uses: solution for administration of
intravenous medications; hydration (may
cause circulatory overload, dilutional
hyponatremia or hypokalemia, or water
intoxication if infused over a prolonged
period of time).

b. 10%, 20%, or 50% *(hypertonic)*
▶ Daily adult requirement: same as for 5%
▶ Uses: treatment of hyperkalemia (may
cause dilutional hypokalemia or
hyponatremia if infused over a prolonged
period of time without electrolytes); to
provide nutrition (insulin may need to be
added to prevent overtaxing the pancreas).

2. Sodium chloride (NaCl)

a. Isotonic (0.9%)
▶ Uses: extracellular fluid replacement (may
cause electrolyte imbalances if used
exclusively for a prolonged period of time);
flushing (TPN lines; before and after
incompatible medications); initiating and
terminating blood transfusions; treatment

of metabolic alkalosis (overhydration may cause acidosis)

▸ May cause hyponatremia, circulatory overload, or hypokalemia if large amounts are infused for prolonged periods of time.

b. Hypotonic (0.2% and 0.45% NaCl)

▸ Uses: as an electrolyte replenisher and for hydration

▸ May produce water intoxication and cerebral edema if infused over an extended period of time.

c. Hypertonic (3% and 5% NaCl)

▸ Uses: replacement for severe sodium losses; treatment for dilutional hyponatremia and edema

▸ May produce cellular dehydration if infused over an extended period of time.

3. Dextrose and sodium chloride combined

a. 5% dextrose with 0.9% NaCl (D₅/0.9)

▸ Uses: extracellular fluid replacement; prevent catabolism (formation of ketones) with loss of potassium and intracellular fluid.

b. 2.5% or 5% dextrose together with 0.2% or 0.45% NaCl

▸ Uses: for hydration; to promote diuresis in dehydrated patients or to assess kidney function.

4. Electrolyte solution (lactated Ringer's)

▸ Uses: extracellular fluid replacement (may produce circulatory overload if infused over a prolonged period of time); treatment of mild acidosis

▸ Contraindicated for patients with cardiac dysfunction or liver disease, or severe metabolic acidosis or alkalosis.

CHAPTER 18

Parenteral nutrition, lipid emulsions, and Hickman/Broviac catheters

Total parenteral nutrition (TPN)—also known as hyperalimentation—and lipid-emulsion feeding are likely to be long-term regimens. Furthermore, TPN and lipid solutions are breeding grounds for microorganisms. Thus, extra care should be taken to observe strict aseptic technique in preparing, handling, and administering TPN and lipid solutions. TPN should be prepared under a laminar-flow hood by aseptic methods and used as soon as possible.

A. TOTAL PARENTERAL NUTRITION (TPN)

1. Indications for use

a. Patients with pathological conditions necessitating high caloric and protein requirements. Such patients would include those with the following:

- Burns
- Multiple systems trauma

▸ Acute renal failure
▸ Ulcerative colitis
▸ Crohn's disease
▸ Postoperative debilitation.

b. Patients unable to ingest food. Such patients would include those with:

▸ Crohn's disease with obstruction
▸ Esophageal or gastric carcinoma with upper GI obstruction
▸ Paralytic ileus.

c. Patients who refuse to eat. They include:

▸ Psychiatric patients with depression or anorexia nervosa
▸ Geriatric patients.

2. Duration of therapy

Duration of TPN is totally dependent on the individual patient's overall condition, and the extent and nature of injury or disease. TPN may be given over a short period of time (7 to 10 days) or therapy may extend for a period of several years.

3. Venipuncture

a. Location. TPN is administered through a central vein—most often the subclavian but sometimes the jugulars or femorals. Occasionally a long-line catheter is inserted through a peripheral vein, such as the cephalic, that connects with a central vein.

b. Method. In most institutions, central venipuncture is regarded as a surgical procedure and is performed by a physician or specially trained RN. The catheter-through-needle (CTN) device is inserted under local anesthesia. Before the TPN infusion is started, the patient must be X-rayed to be sure the catheter is correctly placed. To keep the vein open during the X-ray procedure, a standard IV solution—normal (0.9%) saline or 5% dextrose in water—is infused slowly.

c. Complications. Complications occur more frequently with central line placements than with peripheral line insertions. The complications include:

► Pneumothorax
► Hemothorax
► Air embolism
► Thoracic duct injury
► Infection
► Hematoma
► Catheter embolism
► Brachial plexus injury.

Patients should be observed closely during and immediately following a central line placement for signs and symptoms of possible complications.

4. Equipment

► Normal saline or 5% dextrose in water
► TPN solution
► IV tubing with 0.22-μm filter
► Plain lidocaine (Xylocaine), 1% to 2%
► 18-gauge (or larger) CTN device
► Sterile syringe with 25-gauge needle
► Povidone-iodine solution
► Alcohol wipes
► Antimicrobial ointment
► Sterile gloves
► Tincture of benzoin
► Gauze bandage (2 × 2s and 4 × 4s) or transparent dressing
► Tape
► Sterile scissors

- Suture material and surgical needle as requested
- Sterile drapes
- Infusion pump or volume controller.

5. Approaching the patient

Explain the procedure to the patient and try to answer any questions or concerns he/she may have about the procedure. Make sure your patient also understands the following points:

- How to perform the Valsalva maneuver ("take a deep breath, hold it, and bear down with your mouth closed")
- That the position of the catheter will be verified by X-ray
- That an infusion pump or volume controller will be used (when true)
- That freedom of movement may be limited
- That the dressing must be kept clean and dry.

6. Assisting with subclavian venipuncture

- If necessary, clip or shave chest hair
- Place a rolled bath towel or blanket vertically between the patient's shoulder blades
- If your institution requires it, place a mask on the patient
- Place the patient in the Trendelenburg position, with the head turned away from the venipuncture site and the arms straight down at the sides
- Don sterile gloves and mask
- Holding a sterile gauze sponge with sterile clamps, scrub an area 5 to 6 inches around the insertion site with povidone-iodine (change the sponge two or three times)
- Allow the povidone-iodine to dry for at least two minutes
- Place sterile drapes around the site

- Have sterile gloves and mask ready for the physician
- Wipe the top of the anesthetic bottle with alcohol and invert the bottle for the physician
- While the physician is injecting the anesthetic, spike the bottle/bag of 5% dextrose in water or normal saline, hang it, and prime the tubing (see Chapter 6)
- As the physician connects the tubing to the catheter, help the patient perform the Valsalva maneuver (if the patient is unconscious, place your hands just below the diaphragm and press firmly)
- After the physician has connected the tubing and sutured the catheter in place, start the infusion at a slow rate.

7. Dressing
- The venipuncture site should be kept clean and dry at all times
- Clean the area with alcohol swabs from the center of the site to the periphery
- Clean the area with povidone-iodine swabs from the center of the site to the periphery
- Apply an antimicrobial ointment (e.g., povidone-iodine) to the insertion site, if required by hospital policy
- Place a small (2 × 2) sterile gauze sponge over the insertion site (a small slit may be made in the sponge to accommodate the catheter)
- Place a larger (4 × 4) sterile gauze sponge over the smaller one
- Make sure the needle cover is fastened firmly, if the central-line catheter being used calls for one
- Apply a protective dressing solution to all areas around the gauze dressing where tape will be applied to the skin

▶ Allow the protective dressing solution to dry
▶ Tape the gauze pad on all sides to form an occlusive dressing; a sterile transparent dressing may be used in place of the gauze sponges and occlusive dressing
▶ Loop the tubing and secure it with tape
▶ Label the dressing with the date of insertion
▶ Chart the procedure and any pertinent observations in the patient's record.

8. Starting the TPN

After the catheter's position has been verified by X-ray, you should be ready to start the TPN infusion. The solution should have been kept at room temperature for one hour; never use solution directly from the refrigerator.

▶ Remove the protective cap from the TPN bottle and wipe the stopper with alcohol
▶ Take down the 5% dextrose or normal saline bottle, clamp off the tubing, and pull out the spike
▶ Insert the spike in the TPN bottle and hang it
▶ Adjust the flow rate.

9. Charting

On the patient's chart, note this information:

▶ Size and length of the catheter, date and time it was inserted, by whom, vein used, and type or number of TPN solution
▶ Instructions given to the patient
▶ Patient's reaction to the procedure
▶ X-ray confirmation of catheter placement
▶ Any difficulties encountered
▶ Fluid intake and output initiated.

10. Monitoring the patient

a. Complications of TPN.

Because of the danger of contamination, the invasiveness of the catheter, the high glucose concentration and electrolyte composition of the TPN solution, and the large amounts infused, many serious complications are possible. Additional complications may be introduced by the practice of giving supplemental insulin to process the large amounts of glucose in the TPN solution. Therefore, it's essential to observe the patient for developments such as:

- Blood glucose >200 mg/dl—hyperglycemia
- Urine glucose over 1 + —hyperglycemia, osmotic diuresis
- Rapid pulse, elevated temperature, sweating—hypoglycemia
- Elevated temperature, redness, pain, oozing—infection (catheter-associated septicemia should always be considered in the differential diagnosis of fever)
- Swelling around the insertion site, face, or neck—infiltration or venous thrombosis
- Edema, sweating, weakness, restlessness, rapid breathing, pallor, flushing, cramps, other symptoms—electrolyte or acid-base imbalance
- Distended veins in neck, arm, and hands, elevated blood pressure—fluid overload
- Increased BUN (negative nitrogen balance)—hyperglycemic, hyperosmotic nonketotic acidosis (inadequate caloric intake resulting in protein catabolism)
- Weight loss—undernutrition
- Labored breathing, pain in the chest—air embolism.

b. Documentation. Follow your institution's policy in recording the following observations in the patient's chart:

- Vital signs—every four to eight hours
- Urinary sugar, acetone, and specific gravity—every six to eight hours (use Clinistix or Testape, not Clinitest, if the patient is on an antibiotic)
- Body weight—daily
- Fluid intake and output
- Electrolytes, BUN, creatinine, blood sugar, and other blood chemistry as ordered.

11. Dressing and tubing changes

a. Frequency. Change the dressing every 48 hours unless a transparent dressing is used (this may be changed on a weekly basis). Replace the administration set every 24 hours. A 0.22-micron filter should be used on all TPN infusions. The tubing is changed frequently to safeguard against sepsis due to buildup of microorganisms on the inner surface.

b. Procedure. Procedure for dressing and tubing changes is essentially the same as for the initial setup and dressing. When you remove the dressing, carefully inspect the site and surrounding skin for leakage, oozing, redness, swelling, and general condition. Examine the old dressing for evidence of blood, pus, or TPN fluid.

c. Precautions
- Use sterile, no-touch technique, and don a mask and sterile gloves
- Make the change at the catheter-tubing junction as quickly as possible, while the

patient performs the Valsalva maneuver (to help prevent an air embolism), and with head turned in the opposite direction of the site (to prevent contamination of the site).

12. Additional precautions

▸ Keep the dressing dry

▸ Keep the flow rate constant (less than 10% change in an eight-hour period is recommended). If set too fast to "catch up," it may throw the patient into hyperglycemia or osmotic diuresis; if set too slow to "catch up" on time, it could throw the patient into hypoglycemia or insulin shock

▸ Never discontinue TPN therapy abruptly. The rapid decrease in the patient's blood sugar may cause hypoglycemia or insulin shock. Wean the patient down slowly over a period of several hours or hang a 5% or 10% dextrose solution for approximately eight hours prior to discontinuing the infusion entirely

▸ Don't routinely draw blood through the TPN catheter; use another route

▸ Don't piggyback any medication or solution through a TPN catheter.*

B. LIPID EMULSIONS

Lipid emulsions are considered isotonic and therefore may be infused either peripherally or through a central line. They may be administered alone or in conjunction with an amino acid solution. Because lipid emulsions are a colloidal suspension,

---

*The guidelines issued by the Centers for Disease Control state: "In an effort to avoid unnecessary contamination, the hyperalimentation system should not be used to measure the central venous pressure, administer blood products or 'piggyback' medications, or obtain blood samples." Some institutions follow more liberal policies, however.

they should *never* be delivered through a filter, nor should they be shaken vigorously.

1. Purpose
Lipid emulsions may be given:

► To meet caloric needs when the patient can't tolerate some component of the TPN solution— for example, a diabetic who can't handle the 25% to 50% glucose
► To augment TPN therapy and provide additional calories without appreciably increasing the total fluid volume. Lipid emulsions may be piggybacked into a TPN line, using a large-bore needle, if *strict* aseptic technique is used and your institution's policy permits
► To prevent fatty acid deficiencies
► To increase general nutritional status and assist with the absorption of fat-soluble vitamins.

2. Contraindications
Lipid emulsions may be contraindicated for patients who suffer from:

► Severe hepatic or pulmonary disease
► A bone marrow dyscrasia
► A blood coagulation defect caused by a decreased platelet count
► Hyperlipemia.

3. Equipment
► Bottle of lipid emulsion
► Vented tubing
► Alcohol wipes
► 18- or 20-gauge needle
► Tape.

4. Procedure
A lipid emulsion is generally administered through a primary line.

- Let the emulsion stand for 30 minutes after it has been refrigerated
- Examine the bottle for inconsistencies of color or texture (don't shake the bottle)
- Wipe the stopper of the bottle with alcohol
- Close the regulator clamp on the IV administration set
- Insert the spike into the stopper
- Prime the tubing
- Remove the protective cap from the adapter on the administration set and attach the adapter to the hub of the intravenous catheter device
- Regulate the flow rate.

If the lipid emulsion is to be utilized as a piggyback infusion, follow the preceding steps up through "Prime the tubing," then:

- Attach the 18- or 20-gauge needle to the secondary tubing on the lipid emulsion
- Hang the bottle of lipid emulsion higher than the primary solution
- Wipe the piggyback port on the primary line with alcohol
- Insert the needle (be sure there are *no* filters in the line or that you have piggybacked the lipid emulsion *below* the filter)
- Regulate the rate of flow.

Regardless of the method of administration, lipid emulsions should always be started slowly and the patient observed closely for possible reactions, particularly in the first 30 minutes. If no reactions are noted, the rate may be increased. Be sure to:

- Label the bottle and tubing appropriately
- Chart the procedure and any pertinent observations in the patient's record
- Never add any fluid or medications to the lipid emulsion.

5. Monitoring the patient

a. Complications of lipid-emulsion feeding.

Infusion at too fast a rate can cause fatty acid overload. The rate of administration should not exceed 500 ml in four hours. Patients may also experience adverse reactions to the lipid emulsion itself. Immediate signs of an adverse reaction include:

▸ Elevated temperature
▸ Flushing, sweating
▸ Nausea and vomiting
▸ Headache
▸ Chest and back pains
▸ Labored breathing.

A patient who tolerates a lipid emulsion over a short period may still develop complications over several days' duration:

▸ Enlarged liver, jaundice
▸ Enlarged spleen, bleeding
▸ Focal seizures
▸ Peptic ulcer
▸ Hyperlipemia
▸ Thrombocytopenia.

b. Documentation.

Follow your institution's policy in recording the following observations in the patient's chart:

▸ Temperature—every four to eight hours
▸ Fluid intake and output
▸ Body weight—daily
▸ Caloric intake—daily
▸ Serum turbidity (fatty acid clearance)
▸ Hepatic function tests for patients receiving lipid emulsions for prolonged periods
▸ Other studies as ordered.

6. Changing bottles and tubing

a. Frequency. Use a new tubing every time you hang a new bottle of lipid emulsion. If you're not going to give another bottle right away, remove the catheter/needle or convert the site to a heparin lock. If you're going to start another bottle immediately, simply connect the new tubing to the hub of the catheter/needle after the tubing has been primed. Discard any remaining emulsion in the discontinued line.

b. Procedure. The procedure for intermittent infusion is the same as that for starting an infusion, except that you would connect the line to the PRN (heparin) adapter.

C. PERIPHERAL PARENTERAL NUTRITION (PPN)

Peripheral parenteral nutrition (PPN) is the peripheral administration of isotonic amino acids with balanced electrolyte, vitamin, and mineral additives. These solutions may be administered alone or in conjunction with dextrose (not to exceed 10% when given peripherally) and lipid emulsions.

1. Purpose

PPN provides nutritional support for patients with little or no oral intake for periods of short duration (10 to 14 days). For prolonged periods of inadequate nutritional intake, TPN should be considered. Patients receiving PPN:

▸ Should be in relatively good nutritional status
▸ Should not anticipate a significant increase in their nutritional needs.

2. Equipment
▸ Bottle of amino acid solution
▸ Tubing
▸ Alcohol wipe
▸ Tape.

3. Procedure
The procedure for administering an amino acid solution is the same as that for administering any primary solution (see Chapters 8 and 9).

4. Monitoring the patient
The patient's nutritional status should be assessed frequently to assure that the solutions being delivered are adequate to meet his/her needs. Serum glucose, BUN, and creatinine levels should be checked periodically to assist in verifying the patient's nutritional status.

D. HICKMAN/BROVIAC CATHETERS

Hickman/Broviac catheters are central-line catheters (with one or two lumens) and should be treated with the same care and precautions given any central line. The main differences between these catheters and other central-line catheters are:

▸ The manner in which they are placed—placement is a surgical procedure done by a physician in the operating room with a tunneling up through the subcutaneous tissue for insertion of the catheter into the subclavian, cephalic, or internal or external jugular vein
▸ The location of the exit site—the exit site for this type of catheter is generally located either to the right or left of the midsternal area. This location facilitates teaching the patient self-maintenance and self-care

- Duration of placement—they are generally placed on patients requiring long-term drug therapy and/or long-term TPN therapy (oncology patients, patients with inflammatory bowel disease, etc.) and may be left in place for several years
- Flushing procedure—since these catheters are frequently capped, they don't need to have a continuous infusion, but they do need to be flushed periodically, when not in use, with a heparinized solution. The concentration of heparin solution used and the frequency of flushing will vary in policy from one institution to another (3 to 5 ml of 1:100 or 1:1,000 units of heparin/saline flush solution are frequently used, and the catheters are usually flushed from one to three times per day when not in use, according to specified protocol).

Some advantages of a Hickman/Broviac catheter are:

- The patient may go home with the catheter, after learning the principles and technique of self-care, and resume his/her maximum level of functioning
- Blood samples may be drawn from the catheter, reducing the number of required venipunctures
- If the catheter is a double-lumen type, different medications, or TPN and a medication, may be infused simultaneously
- The catheter has a Dacron cuff, located approximately 30 to 36 cm from the distal end, which helps to reduce the risk of infection from bacteria migrating along the skin tract.

CHAPTER 19

Infection control in IV therapy

The preceding chapters have mentioned, in an incidental way, the practical steps necessary to avoid infection. This chapter summarizes the ways in which IV systems can become contaminated with microorganisms and suggests measures for preventing nosocomial infections resulting from IV therapy.

A. SOURCES OF INFECTION

1. Intrinsic and extrinsic

a. Intrinsic. Intrinsic sources of contamination are those present in the IV equipment before unpackaging and use:

- ▸ Cracks in bottles
- ▸ Punctures in bags
- ▸ Contaminated solution or blood
- ▸ Administration set
- ▸ Venipuncture device

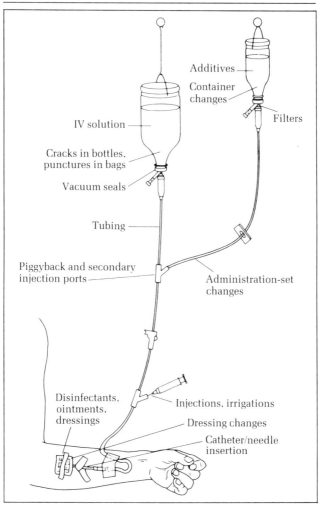

Figure 19-1 *Intrinsic and extrinsic sources of contamination*

▶ Ointment
▶ Gauze, tape, etc., used for dressing.

b. Extrinsic. Extrinsic sources of contamination are those introduced in setting up and running an infusion:

▶ Additives
▶ Attachment of the bottle/bag to the administration set
▶ Infusion pump/volume controller or volume-control chamber
▶ Piggybacks
▶ Secondary infusions
▶ Add-on filter
▶ Insertion of catheter/needle
▶ Stopcocks
▶ CVP manometer.

The illustration (Figure 19-1) summarizes intrinsic and extrinsic sources of contamination.

2. Patient's skin flora

a. Organisms. The organisms that are most commonly cultured from catheter tips are *Staphylococcus epidermidis*, *S. aureus*, and gram-negative bacilli and enterococci. A similar microbial profile has been observed in cases of catheter-associated septicemia. All these organisms are normal skin flora and therefore should be expected to be present on the skin of hospitalized patients.

b. Mechanisms of contamination. It's been suggested that skin flora gain access to catheter tips in either of two ways:

▶ At the moment of insertion
▶ By migrating along the interface between the catheter and the patient's tissues.

c. Prevention
▶ Thorough cleansing of the patient's skin
▶ Immobilization of catheters/needles
▶ Maintaining the site clean and dry.

3. Hospital personnel

a. Organisms. In addition to the organisms normally present on skin, antibiotic-resistant gram-negative bacteria frequently contaminate the hands of hospital personnel.

b. Mechanisms of contamination
▶ Failure to wash hands sufficiently
▶ Touching portions of IV equipment that should not be touched—e.g., needle and catheter tips, tubing ends, stoppers on bottles/bags
▶ Unnecessary manipulation of IV systems that are running.

c. Prevention
▶ Wash hands vigorously with antimicrobial soap before initiating an infusion, before manipulating the system (e.g., tubing changes), and between patients
▶ Always avoid touch contamination
▶ Don't handle any component of an IV system more than is necessary.

4. Hospital environment

Hospital air, surfaces, and fomites are generally considered not to be significant sources of microbial infection. However, don't expose any portion of an IV system to the air longer than is necessary, and be careful not to let any sterile portion of the system touch a nonsterile surface. Keep all ports on stopcocks covered at all times; stopcocks are a major source of contamination of IV systems. Keep all IV systems as "closed" as possible.

5. The patient

It's been found that the rate of microbial contamination of catheter tips is significantly higher in individuals who present with an infection before IV therapy is begun than in noninfected patients. Take extra care to use aseptic technique with infected patients, both to prevent systemic infection via the IV catheter/needle and to protect yourself and others with whom you come in contact.

6. The IV system

a. Solution. IV solutions, especially those containing glucose, are excellent growth media for various microorganisms. Within 24 hours, *Klebsiella* and other gram-negative bacteria can multiply in glucose-containing IV solutions to levels that are likely to cause clinical sepsis. Reflux of blood into the tubing may provide nutrients that allow additional species to thrive in the solution. Buffering of acidic dextrose solutions with bicarbonate likewise promotes the growth of additional organisms. The Centers for Disease Control make these recommendations for preventing infection:

- ▸ ". . . no intravenous bottle or bag should be left in place for more than 24 hours"
- ▸ Bottles and bags should be closely inspected for the presence of cracks and punctures that are too small to permit leakage but large enough to let bacteria in, and for turbidity and precipitation
- ▸ When there is suspicion that the fluid may be contaminated, the fluid should be cultured and the lot number noted.

b. Administration set. Microorganisms capable of growing in IV solutions can live in IV tubing for days. Even when the infusion is continuous and rapid, bacteria are capable of ascending the tubing and contaminating the IV solution. Therefore, administration sets should be changed at least every 24 to 48 hours, and guarded against contamination at both the proximal and distal ends.

c. Dressings. Dressings, being occlusive, provide a warm, moist environment for bacteria and fungi. Use of topical antibacterial preparations is likely to promote overgrowth of the yeast *Candida* and various resistant bacterial strains. Therefore, use an agent—povidone-iodine—that kills not only bacteria but also fungi, protozoa, and yeasts. Change the dressing and apply new povidone-iodine solution or ointment every 24 hours. If a sterile transparent dressing is used, it may remain in place until the catheter/needle is changed (48 to 72 hours) as long as the site remains clean and dry. If the dressing becomes wet, soiled, or otherwise contaminated, the area needs to be cleansed and new povidone-iodine solution or ointment and dressing applied.

d. Catheter/needle. Stainless-steel winged needles are thought by some to produce less infection than CON devices, but there is information refuting this claim. Winged needles tend to cause infiltration and have to be replaced more frequently. The Centers for Disease Control recommend changing catheters/needles every 48 to 72 hours.

7. Blood

Septic shock resulting from transfusion of blood heavily contaminated with gram-negative bacteria is reported to carry a high mortality rate. The responsible organisms in these studies were mostly psychrophilic species, including *Pseudomonas* and coliform species. Fortunately, clinical infection from contaminated blood is quite rare. Four precautions help prevent infection:

- ► Use blood and blood products as soon as possible after they're taken from the refrigerator
- ► Discard the entire administration set after the transfusion
- ► Don't allow blood to hang for over four hours
- ► Avoid touch contamination of the blood and infusion system.

B. MANAGEMENT OF SUSPECTED INFECTION

No matter how much care is taken, infections will occasionally develop as a result of IV therapy. Phlebitis at the puncture site is present in more than half the cases of infusion-associated septicemia, so phlebitis should immediately bring the IV system to mind when a patient develops a systemic infection (see Chapter 15). The IV system should also be suspected in the absence of noticeable phlebitis, especially if the catheter/needle has been in place for over 72 hours.

1. Determining whether septicemia is due to IV infusion

a. Obtaining culture specimens

- ► Culture IV sites and systems according to your hospital's policies and procedures. Be careful not to contaminate the specimens during the collection process

► Carefully examine the insertion site; if it shows any sign of infection, take a culture sample

► Obtain blood samples from two separate venipuncture sites if the patient is febrile

► If possible, obtain blood culture specimens through the catheter to determine whether an infected thrombus is present

► Remove the entire infusion system, including the catheter/needle, and start a new infusion at another site (preferably the opposite limb)

► Send a sample of any fluid remaining in the system to the lab

► Send a culture of any pus or exudate from the site to the lab

► Cut the distal 1/3 to 1/2 of the catheter with sterile scissors, place it in the appropriate medium (according to the hospital's policies and procedures), and send it to the lab.

b. Criteria for determining whether an infection is due to IV infusion

► Culture positive for organisms at the insertion site

► Positive catheter-tip culture, with more than 15 colonies, if clinical evidence of infection is also present

► Purulent drainage at the insertion site.

Inflammation (redness, tenderness, swelling, warmth) of the insertion site without evidence of purulent drainage or cellulitis should not be regarded as infection unless a catheter-tip culture is positive.

2. Treatment

The entire IV system (cannula, administration set, and fluid) is to be changed immediately if purulent thrombophlebitis, cellulitis, or IV-related bacteremia is strongly suspected or verified by blood cultures, and all materials and the site are to be cultured appropriately. For phlebitis without signs of infection, the site should be changed immediately to the opposite limb. Fortunately, infusion-associated bacteremias and fungemias often resolve spontaneously once the offending infusion system is removed. However, appropriate antibiotics should be given to the patient if clinical signs of infection or positive cultures persist.

3. Documentation

a. Suspect products. Record the nature and lot number of any suspect product. If evidence suggests contamination at the time of manufacture, local health authorities and the Food and Drug Administration should be notified.

b. Culture specimens. Label each specimen with the following information:

- Patient's name and ID number
- Room number
- Date and time
- Site from which the specimen was taken.

c. Charting. Record the date, time, and site of all culture specimens. When results come back from the lab, record them.

d. IV therapy statistical records. Record the patient's name, ID number, room number, date, time, site, and lab result for each culture specimen you take.

C. CONTAMINATED NEEDLES

1. Disposal

After beginning an infusion, the contaminated needle/stylet should be discarded in a puncture-proof container specific for that purpose. Never throw needles into a trash can or leave them uncapped where others may be stuck by them.

2. Injury

Injury from a contaminated needle should be reported promptly to your supervisor or the employee health nurse for investigation and treatment.

CHAPTER 20

Legal, religious, and psychological aspects of IV therapy

A. LAWS AND REGULATIONS

1. Personnel

a. State laws. Different states have different laws concerning who may administer IV therapy. Certification authority for any nursing function rests with the state's board of nurses and the state's nurse practice act. Responsibility for this function may be delegated to other groups such as the state's nurses' association or the National Intravenous Therapy Association (NITA), or may be handled by the state's board of consumer affairs for non-nursing personnel.

b. Institutional regulations. Within each state, different institutions may have different policies regarding who may administer IV therapy. Increasingly, such policies are detailed in written IV manuals. In addition to specifying who can give IV infusions, there may be policies governing procedures such as blood transfusion, placement of central lines, and injection of IV medications.

2. IV manual

Your institution's IV manual probably contains detailed descriptions of the following:

▶ Personnel—who is allowed to perform what procedures
▶ The equipment to be used in each type of procedure
▶ Verifying patients' identities
▶ Handwashing requirements
▶ Procedures for prepping patients
▶ How to perform each IV procedure
▶ Disposal of used IV equipment
▶ How to use specialized equipment, and who is permitted to do so
▶ Infusion times for various medications
▶ Special instructions for various areas such as the ICU/CCU and emergency department.

3. Charting

Only complete and accurate records will serve the medicolegal needs of your patients, the hospital, physicians, hospital staff, and you.

a. What to chart. No matter how routine or insignificant something may seem to be, you should write it in a patient's permanent record. Legally speaking, if something is *not charted*, it is considered *not done*.

b. Erasures. A patient's record is a legal document. Write everything in ink. Never use correction fluid or erase anything you write there. If you make an error, ink a line through it, write "error" above it, include the date and your initials, and then insert the correct information.

c. Objectivity. Keep your charting as objective as possible. Use quotation marks for direct quotes and statements of opinion by others. Attribute all quotations. Use words like "appeared" and "alleged" when writing about things that aren't proven.

4. Legal liability

a. Responsibility. You are responsible for your own acts and can be sued for negligence if you fail to act in accordance with the standards set by your institution and the state board of nurses. Standards of practice, as stated by professional organizations and other health-care providers, are frequently utilized in determining the standard of care in any given area for a particular service or specialty.

b. Errors of omission. Errors of omission can be just as detrimental as errors of commission. Failure to act prudently, in accordance with your knowledge and training, could result in a legal judgment against you.

c. Good Samaritan laws. You cannot be found liable if you aid a person in distress unless you:

- Exceed the limits of your training
- Commit an act of gross negligence
- Charge for your services.

In giving emergency care, you'll decrease your chances of being sued if you take the following steps:

- Keep up your certification, skills, and knowledge

- Defer to the person on the scene who has the highest level of training
- Follow up patients if you were the person in charge during the emergency.

d. Patients' rights. Patients have certain rights that must be considered and protected. Many states have incorporated patients' rights into some form of legislative or administrative code. These "rights" frequently include the following, but check with your state authorities to determine your exact obligations concerning patients' rights in your area.

- Considerate and respectful care without regard to sex or cultural, economic, educational, or religious background
- Knowledge of the patient's primary-care physician and information from his physician about his illness, proposed course of treatment, and prognosis
- Receipt of information regarding any proposed treatment and/or specific procedures, and active participation in the decisions regarding the patient's own care—including the right to refuse any treatment or procedure
- Confidential treatment and privacy concerning all communications and records regarding the patient's medical care
- Ability to leave the hospital "against medical advice" (AMA), unless being detained on a legal hold
- Knowledge concerning all hospital rules and regulations that apply to the patient's conduct

- ▸ Reasonable responses to reasonable questions regarding the patient's care and requests for service
- ▸ Being advised if the hospital or physician proposes to engage in or perform human experimentation affecting the patient's care or treatment (the patient has the right to refuse to participate in such research projects)
- ▸ Being informed of the patient's continuing health-care requirements following his discharge
- ▸ Examination of the patient's hospital bill and receipt of an explanation of the costs regardless of source of payment.

B. RELIGIOUS BELIEFS

1. Respect
Patients have the right to receive respect for all their religious beliefs. Before giving IV therapy, explain to the patient what you're going to do, and why. If the patient has a concern based on religious persuasion, a simple explanation may clear up misunderstandings and reassure him/her. If, after a thorough explanation, the patient refuses to undergo treatment or a procedure, that refusal must be respected unless it's overruled by a court decision. Notify the patient's physician of the refusal and document your actions in the patient's record.

2. Objectivity
Never let your own religious beliefs affect your attitude toward a patient.

3. Certain religious beliefs concerning IV therapy and medical treatment

a. Jehovah's Witnesses. Members of this sect do not believe in blood transfusion or the administration of any blood product, including plasma and albumin. These individuals will usually cooperate if assured that an IV doesn't contain any blood product. In a test case in 1980, a Jehovah's Witness accepted infusion of an artificial product capable of transporting oxygen.

b. Christian Scientists. Christian Scientists attain various levels of religious experience. Those who feel they've reached a high level of "science awareness" may refuse to accept any form of medical assistance.

c. Other beliefs. Some people believe that admission of pain or debility is a human weakness and reflects lack of religious faith. Others believe that by enduring pain they can transcend their bodies and attain a higher state of being in the afterlife. Still others believe that pain and suffering are God's punishment for their sins. Individuals with beliefs of these sorts may refuse IV therapy and other medical treatment.

C. PSYCHOLOGY IN IV THERAPY

Trauma, disease, and hospital equipment are everyday encounters for you, but they may be new and very frightening experiences for patients. In addition to the pain, discomfort, and debility caused by the patient's physical condition, the experience of being in a hospital and of losing control of one's life and of one's individuality may produce a great deal of psychological stress.

1. Emotional crisis

a. Types of crisis. A crisis is an emotionally significant event or radical change in one's life. There are two types of medical crisis:

- Expected—when the patient has been ill for some time
- Unexpected—when sudden trauma or illness strikes.

b. Stages of a crisis

- Impact—usually seen by emergency personnel
- Recoil—usually seen by hospital personnel
- Post-trauma—seen by hospital personnel and by the patient's family after discharge.

c. Resolution. An emotional crisis is usually resolved by one of the following approaches:

- Problem solving
- Redefinition
- Adoption of a defense mechanism: denial, rationalization, etc.

2. Persons involved in a crisis

Three categories of people are involved in an emotional crisis:

- The person experiencing the crisis—the patient
- Significant others—family, close friends
- Onlookers—emergency and hospital personnel, casual friends, interested bystanders.

Your task is to meet the immediate, life-threatening needs of the patient and to provide calm, objective support for the patient and his/her significant others.

3. Reactions to crisis and pain

a. Individual coping mechanisms. Everyone learns various ways of coping with situations that are frightening, painful, unexpected, embarrassing, suspenseful, or otherwise uncomfortable. To a certain extent, ethnic, cultural, religious, and socioeconomic factors determine how individuals cope with crisis and pain. A few commonly utilized mechanisms for coping are:

▶ *Conversion:* Conversion operates wholly on an unconscious level and allows the patient to convert strong emotional conflicts into physical symptoms (hysterical paralysis, headaches, GI symptoms, etc.)

▶ *Denial:* A patient may simply reject the fact of his illness or crisis. This is seen fairly often on medical and surgical units, and could have serious consequences for the patient with a major health problem. Patients coping through denial often retreat into themselves and become quite withdrawn

▶ *Displacement:* The transference of emotion from one object, situation, or idea to another (e.g., being angry with "God" or "fate" because of a particular crisis or disease, and yelling at and blaming the nurse or doctor for the problem)

▶ *Identification or introjection:* Acceptance of a person or idea, feeling as though it is a part of one's self

▶ *Projection:* The act of attributing unacceptable faults, failures, thoughts, or activities within the person to others in order to protect "self." This is frequently exhibited in angry shouting, inappropriate accusations, and demanding behavior

▶ *Rationalization:* A method of self-deception, it is simply finding a logical reason for the things one wants to do

▶ *Reaction formation:* The process of overcompensating for a negative feeling or activity by overdeveloping the opposite behavior. Someone who is *overly* sweet and polite may be attempting to disguise an underlying hostility. Inappropriate humor or joking may be covering up underlying fear

▶ *Regression:* A common form of coping frequently found in hospitals, regression occurs when the patient reverts to previous patterns of behavior that were successful in earlier stages of development (temper tantrums, crying, attachment, etc.)

▶ *Repression:* A patient actively forces unpleasant or unacceptable facts or experiences into his/her unconscious mind. The facts and/or experiences really *can't* be remembered. Repression operates wholly on an unconscious level

▶ *Sublimation:* The act of substituting an acceptable activity (e.g., chewing gum) for an unacceptable one (e.g., smoking)

▶ *Symbolization:* A mental mechanism of the subconscious in which one idea or object stands for another.

b. Physiological effects. The physiological changes produced by the patient's physical condition may be made better or worse by his/her emotional reaction to the stress of crisis and pain—for example, loss of appetite due to depression or venospasms due to fear.

c. Reactivation of unresolved emotions. The stress of crisis and pain may bring to the surface unresolved fears, anxieties, or problems that the patient had previously managed to suppress. This response is especially likely to happen when the patient subconsciously perceives a similarity between a stressful incident in the past and the present crisis. Bear this in mind when a patient appears disoriented or displays inappropriate behavior; he/she may be reliving a traumatic episode from the past.

4. Perception of pain

The degree and quality of pain perceived by the patient are as variable as other sensory perceptions. Even more variable may be the degree and manner of patients' expression of pain.

5. Your treatment of the patient

a. Acceptance. Accept the patient and family as they are. Acceptance doesn't mean approval. Acceptance of the present situation also doesn't mean that you won't accept changes in emotional outlook and behavior when they occur.

b. Listening. Let the patient and significant others ventilate their thoughts and feelings, both overt and covert. Sometimes covert signals (inflections in the voice, gestures, body language, etc.) are more significant in uncovering the "truth" about thoughts and feelings than is the overtly spoken word. *All behavior has meaning.* It is important that we develop a sensitivity to others' thoughts and feelings (both covert and overt) in order to understand the meaning behind the behavior. If we are to be effective in helping others to cope with their present problems and situations, and to proceed beyond the crisis of the moment to a healthy resolution and acceptable behavior, we must be "tuned in" to them by watching, listening, evaluating, and understanding the true essence of their thoughts and feelings.

c. Objectivity. Keep your own feelings out of your relationships with patients. Watch not only what you say but also how you say it. Be friendly and courteous; don't be afraid to be human and show that you care. Empathy— an *objective* awareness and insight into the feelings, emotions, and behavior of others, and their meaning and significance—is an integral part of caring. If you can't be objective in dealing with a particular patient, ask someone else to care for him/her if at all possible. If you don't, chances are that you will probably reveal to that patient, in a covert manner, your dislike for him/her. This may have a negative effect not only on the patient but on you and other members of the health-care team.

d. Discretion. You should never discuss a patient's condition with him/her or with the family. Never pass judgment or imply any deprecation of other health personnel or previous treatment in front of a patient or family. Be careful not to discuss a patient's problems or condition in public places where family members, friends, or visitors may hear you (e.g., elevators, cafeteria, lobby).

6. Minimizing anxiety

You can do a great deal to minimize patients' fears just by following these simple steps.

a. Explain. Always tell the patient who you are and what you're going to do. Encourage questions; the patient may have misconceptions about IV therapy, learned from television or other sources.

b. Be friendly, courteous, and supportive.

c. Prepare equipment out of sight. Try to do as much preliminary preparation as possible out of the patient's sight and hearing. This usually helps minimize anxiety concerning the appearance and use of equipment.

Bibliography

Anderson AO, Yardley JH: Demonstration of Candida in blood smears. *N Engl J Med* 286:108, 1972

Ansel HC, Gifandet MP: Change in pH of infusion solutions upon mixing with blood. *JAMA* 218:1052, 1971

Banks DC, Tates DB, Cawdrey HM, et al: Infection from intravenous catheters. *Lancet* 1:443, 1970

Bernard RW, Stahl WM, Chase RM: Subclavian vein catheterizations: A prospective study. II. Infectious complications. *Ann Surg* 173:191, 1971

Boeckman CR, Krill CE Jr: Bacterial and fungal infections complicating parenteral alimentation. *J Pediatr Surg* 5:117, 1970

Bolasny BL, Martin CE, Conkle DM: Careful technique with plastic intravenous catheters. *Surg Gynecol Obstet* 131:1030, 1971

Bolasny BL, Shepard GH, Scott HW, et al: The hazards of intravenous polyethylene catheters in surgical patients. *Surg Gynecol Obstet* 130:342, 1970

Braude AI: Transfusion reactions from contaminated blood, their recognition and treatment. *N Engl J Med* 258:1289, 1958

Braude AI, Carey FJ, Siemienski J: Studies of bacterial transfusion reactions from refrigerated blood: Properties of cold-growing bacteria. *J Clin Invest* 34:311, 1955

Braude AI, Sanford JP, Barlett JE, et al: Effects and clinical significance of bacterial contaminants in transfused blood. *J Lab Clin Med* 39:902, 1952

Brennan MF, O'Connell RC, Rosol JA, et al: The growth of Candida albicans in nutritive solutions given parenterally. *Arch Surg* 103:705, 1971

Brereton RB: Incidence of complications from indwelling venous catheters. *Del Med J* 41:1, 1969

Center for Disease Control: Nosocomial bacteremias associated with intravenous fluid therapy—USA. *Morbid Mortal Weekly Rep* 20, 1971

Chaffee EE, Greisheimer EM: *Basic Physiology and Anatomy*, 3rd ed. Philadelphia: Lippincott, 1974

Cheney FW, Lincol JR: Phlebitis from plastic intravenous catheters. *Anesthesiology* 25:650, 1964

Collins RN, Braun PA, Zinner SH, et al: Risk of local and systemic infections with polyethylene intravenous catheters. *N Engl J Med* 279.340, 1968

Colvin MP, Blogg CE, Savage TM, et al: A safe long-term infusion technique? *Lancet* 2:317, 1972

Corso JA, Agostinelli R, Brandriss MW: Maintenance of venous polyethylene catheters to reduce risk of infection. *JAMA* 210:2075, 1969

Crenshaw CA, Kelly L, Turner RJ, et al: Bacteriologic nature and prevention of contamination to intravenous catheters. *Am J Surg* 123:264, 1972

Crenshaw CA, Kelly L, Turner RJ, et al: Prevention of infection at scalp vein needle insertion during intravenous therapy. *Am J Surg* 124:43, 1972

Duma RJ, Warner JB, Dalton HP: Septicemia from intravenous infusions. *N Engl J Med* 284:257, 1971

Felts SK, Schaffner W, Melly MA, et al: Sepsis caused by contaminated intravenous fluids: Epidemiologic, clinical and laboratory investigation of an outbreak in one hospital. *Ann Intern Med* 77:881, 1972

Fisher EJ, Maki DG, Eisses J, et al: Epidemic septicemias due to intrinsically contaminated infusion products. *Abstr 11th Intersci Conf Antimicrob Agents Chemother (Atlantic City)*, p 20, October 20, 1971

Freeman R, King B: Infective complications of indwelling intravenous catheters and the monitoring of infections by the nitroblue-tetrazolium test. *Lancet* 1:992, 1972

Fuchs PC: Indwelling intravenous polyethylene catheters. Factors influencing the risk of microbial colonization and sepsis. *JAMA* 216:1447, 1971

Fundamentals of Body Water and Electrolytes. Deerfield, Ill: Baxter Laboratories, Division of Travenol Laboratories, Inc., 1974

Glover JL, O'Byrne SA, Jolly I: Infusion catheter sepsis: An increasing threat. *Ann Surg* 173:148, 1971

Goldfarb IW, Yates AP: *Total Parenteral Nutrition Concepts and Methods.* Pittsburgh: Synapse Publications, 1980

Goldmann DA: Prevention of infection in hyperalimentation therapy. *9th Int Cong Nutr (Mexico City)*, Sept 3, 1972

Gray: *Anatomy, Descriptive and Surgical.* Philadelphia: Running Press, 1974

Habibi B, Salmon C: Septic shock from bacterial contamination of transfused blood. *Lancet* 2:830, 1972

Hoshal VL: Intravenous catheters and infection. *Surg Clin North Am* 52:1407, 1972

Insights Into Parenteral Nutrition. Deerfield, Ill: Travenol Laboratories, Inc., 1977

James JD: Bacterial contamination of reserved blood. *Vox Sang* 4:177, 1959

Krauss RN, Albert RF, Kannan MM: Contamination of catheters in the infant. *J Pediatr* 77:965, 1970

Levy RS, Goldstein J, Pressman RS: Value of a topical antibiotic ointment in reducing bacterial colonization of percutaneous venous catheters. *J Albert Einstein Med Cent* 18:67, 1970

Lowenbraun S, Young V, Kenton D, et al: Infection from intravenous "scalp vein" needles in a susceptible population. *JAMA* 212:451, 1970

Maintenance Peripheral Nutrition. Deerfield, Ill: Travenol Laboratories, Inc., 1976

Maki DG, Rhame FS, Goldmann DA, et al: The infection hazard posed by contaminated intravenous infusion fluid. In *Clinical and Laboratory Aspects of Bacteremias—A Symposium* (Sonnenwirth AC, ed). Springfield, Ill: Thomas, 1973

Maki DG, Rhame FS, Mackel DC, et al: Nosocomial septicemias subsequent to contaminated intravenous fluid. *Proc Annu Meet Am Soc Microbiol (Minnesota)*, May 5, 1971

Managing I.V. Therapy. Horsham, Pa: Intermed Communications (Nursing Photobook Service), 1982

Matheney RV, Topalis M: *Psychiatric Nursing*, 5th ed. St. Louis: Mosby, 1970

Mays ET: A microbiological investigation of percutaneous central venous catheters. *South Med J* 65:830, 1972

Meng HC, Wilmore DW: *Fat Emulsions in Parenteral Nutrition.* Chicago: American Medical Association, 1976

Michaels L, Ruebner B: Growth of bacteria in intravenous infusion fluids. *Lancet* 1:772, 1953

Moore FD, Brennan MF: Intravenous feeding. *N Engl J Med* 287:862, 1972

Morgensen JV, Frederiksen W, Jensen JK: Subclavian vein catheterization and infection: A bacteriologic study of 130 catheter insertions. *Scand J Infect Dis* 4:31, 1972

Morton HD: Alcohols. In *Disinfection, Sterilization, and Preservation* (Lawrence CA, Black SS, eds), p 237. Philadelphia: Lea & Febiger, 1968

Norden CW: Application of antibiotic ointment to the site of venous catheterization—A controlled trial. *J Infect Dis* 120:611, 1969

Page BH, Raine G, Jones PF: Thrombophlebitis following intravenous infusions. *Lancet* 2:778, 1952

Plumer A: *Principles and Practice of Intravenous Therapy,* 3rd ed. Boston: Little, Brown, 1982

Pollack M, Charache P, Nieman RE, et al: Factors influencing colonization and antibiotic-resistant patterns of gram-negative bacteria in hospital patients. *Lancet* 2:668, 1972

Sager DP, Bomar SK: *Intravenous Medications: A Guide to Preparation, Administration, and Nursing Management.* Philadelphia: Lippincott, 1980

Salzman TC, Clark JJ, Klemm L: Hand contamination of personnel as a mechanism of cross-infection in nosocomial infection with antibiotic-resistant Escherichia coli and Klebsiella aerobacter. *Antimicrob Agents Chemother* 97, 1967

Sanderson I, Deitel M: Intravenous hyperalimentation without sepsis. *Surg Gynecol Obstet* 136:577, 1973

Selwin S, Ellis H: Skin bacteria and skin disinfection reconsidered. *Br Med J* 1:136, 1972

White JJ, Wallace CK, Burnett LS: Skin disinfection. *Johns Hopkins Med J* 126:169, 1970

Wilmore DW, Groff DB, Bishop HC, et al: Total parenteral nutrition in infants with catastrophic gastrointestinal anomalies. *J Pediatr Surg* 4:181, 1969

Zinner SH, Denny-Brown BC, Braun P, et al: Risk of infection with intravenous indwelling catheters: Effective application of antibiotic ointment. *J Infect Dis* 120:616, 1969

Index

Italicized page numbers denote illustrations or tabulated material.